42nd VLAG thematic m

Folate & age-related disease

October 22, 2004

11:45 - 12:30	Reception & Lunch
12:30 - 12:40	Welcome & introduction *Dr. P. Verhoef, Wageningen Centre for Food Sciences*
12:40 - 13:05	Recent insights in intracellular folate regulation *Dr. M.C. Anguera, Harvard Medical School*
13:05 - 13:30	Cellular function of folate: going beyond homocysteine *Dr. Y.M. Smulders, Vrije University Medical Center*
13:30 - 13:55	Folate and vascular disease: mechanisms and evidence *Dr. M.C. Verhaar, Utrecht University*
13:55 - 14:10	Break
14:10 - 14:35	Folate and neurodegenerative disorders: mechanisms and evidence *Dr. C.E. Teunissen, Vrije University Medical Center*
14:35 - 15:00	Is folic acid fortification effective? *Prof. J. Selhub, Tufts University*
15:00 - 15:10	Perspective of folate research *Dr. P. Verhoef, Wageningen Centre for Food Sciences*
15:10 - 15:45	Break & travel to Aula, Wageningen University
16:00 - 17:30	Ph.D. defense, Folate and age-related disease (Aula) *J. Durga, Wageningen University*

The Graduate School VLAG

Wageningen Centre for Food Sciences

LOCATION Wageningen University, Scheikundegebouw 316, Lecture hall C6
REGISTER before October 15, 2004. Contact ondine.vanderest@wur.nl or 0317-483521

Folate and age-related disease

Promotoren
Prof. dr. ir. Frans J. Kok
Hoogleraar Voeding en Gezondheid
Wageningen Universiteit

Prof. dr. Evert G. Schouten
Hoogleraar Epidemiologie en Preventie
Wageningen Universiteit

Co-promotor
dr. ir. Petra Verhoef
Projectleider
Wageningen Centre for Food Sciences / Wageningen Universiteit

Promotiecommissie
Prof. dr. Willibrord H.L. Hoefnagels
Radboud Universiteit Nijmegen

Prof. dr. Jacob Selhub
Tufts University

Prof. dr. ir. Daan Kromhout
Wageningen Universiteit

Prof. dr. Coen D.A. Stehouwer
Universiteit Maastricht

Dit onderzoek is uitgevoerd binnen de onderzoekschool VLAG.

Jane Durga

Folate and age-related disease

Proefschrift

ter verkrijging van de graad van doctor
op gezag van de rector magnificus
van Wageningen Universiteit,
prof. dr. ir. L. Speelman,
in het openbaar te verdedigen
op vrijdag 22 oktober 2004
des namiddags te vier uur in de Aula

Durga, Jane

Folate and age-related disease
Thesis Wageningen University – with references – with summary in Dutch

ISBN 90 8504 091 4

to my loving family

Abstract

Background Aging is associated with increased risk of cardiovascular and neurodegenerative disorders and an increase in their risk factors, such as decreased concentrations of folate and increased concentrations of homocysteine. The association of folate and homocysteine with age-related disease and, most importantly, the causality needs to be assessed for effective public health policy. The pathogenic mechanisms, which link these risk factors to age-related diseases may include non-specific disease mechanisms such as inflammation.

Methods We investigated the association of folate and homocysteine with cardiovascular disease risk, cognitive performance on a battery of neuropsychological tests and hearing thresholds in middle-aged and elderly men and post-menopausal women using cross-sectional data obtained from the baseline measurements of the FACIT trial. FACIT is an acronym for Folic Acid and Carotid Intima-media Thickness. The FACIT trial investigates the effects of daily folic acid supplementation (0.8 mg/d) for three years on age-related parameters, carotid artery wall thickness and arterial stiffness, cognitive performance and hearing. Furthermore, we investigated whether supplementation with folic acid after one year will lead to a reduction in plasma concentrations of inflammation markers in the final 530 participants of the FACIT trial.

Results Low folate status and high concentrations of homocysteine were associated with increased carotid intima-media thickness, a marker of cardiovascular disease risk. However, the relationships were explained to a great part by conventional risk factors (mean difference between first vs. fourth quartile of erythrocyte folate 0.03 mm, 95% confidence interval -0.002 to 0.06 mm). Neither folate nor homocysteine were associated with carotid distension, a measure of arterial stiffness. Decreased concentrations of erythrocyte folate and increased concentrations of homocysteine were independently associated with poor cognitive performance. The cognitive domains with the greatest variability with age, like memory and speed-related functions, were also the domains with the strongest relation with low folate levels. Unexpectedly, folate, not homocysteine, was directly associated with hearing impairment; however, this association was confined to subjects with the 5,10-methylenetetrahydrofolate reductase (MTHFR) 677C allele. Subjects with the MTHFR 677TT genotype had better cognitive performance and hearing levels than subjects with the CC or CT genotype. Finally, inflammation markers did not respond to one-year folic acid supplementation, despite a 25% decrease in homocysteine concentrations.

Conclusions and implications Increased concentrations of folate, independent of its role in homocysteine-lowering, are weakly associated with decreased risk of cardiovascular disease and better cognitive function, but not with hearing acuity. Further research is required to establish whether these relationships are causal and the mechanism responsible for disease. If faced with the decision whether to fortify the national food chain with folic acid, public health policy makers should wait for the large trials to report their findings on the effects of folic acid—alone or in combination with other B vitamins—on cardiovascular disease and dementia.

"*Folate and age-related disease*," Ph.D. thesis by Jane Durga, Division of Human Nutrition, Wageningen University, Wageningen, October 22, 2004.

Contents

Chapter 1

Let them eat cake

Jane Durga, Petra Verhoef

Division of Human Nutrition, Wageningen University, Wageningen, The Netherlands
Wageningen Centre for Food Sciences, Wageningen, The Netherlands

Submitted

Panacea

Folic acid, the synthetic form of folate, a B vitamin, has been called the leading contender for the panacea of the 21st century.[1] The speed at which folate has reached new heights as a cure-all for many modern day ills is astonishing, even faster than the introduction of sugar to the common man's diet.[2] Lucy Wills, in 1931, reported on a factor in yeast which could correct macrocytic anemia in pregnant women, later revealed to be folate. Macrocytic anemia in patients with celiac disease, idiopathic steatorrhoea, sprue and undernutrition responded better to folic acid, newly synthesized by Bob Stockstad in 1943, than to liver or yeast extracts.[3] The historical context may explain why definitions of folate deficiency are based on abnormal changes in blood such as macrocytic anemia. Since the discovery of folate, low concentrations of folate have been linked to a multitude of diseases and chronic conditions, like vascular disease, dementia and age-related hearing loss, either as a cause or a consequence.[4,5]

Folate from food

Folate is present almost ubiquitously in natural foods, but still many adults do not consume enough folate to meet the dietary reference intake. The estimated folate intake in Dutch aged 20 to 65 years is approximately ~200-250 μg/d, lower than the dietary reference intake of 300 μg of folate per day.[6] One can achieve adequate folate status eating a diet high in folate-rich foods such as fruits and vegetables.[7-10] Poor dietary habits e.g. diets high in refined grains, high-fat dairy products and red meat rather than fruits and vegetables, whole grains and poultry, may help explain low dietary folate intake and low folate concentrations.[11-18]

Dietary patterns are known to change with age, and aging has been associated with lower folate intake and low folate concentrations.[19-21] In addition to poor dietary habits, aging may influence one's folate metabolism. With increasing age, the activity of enzymes involved in folate metabolism may decrease and the incidence of malabsorptive intestinal disease, like atrophic gastritis increases. Furthermore, folate metabolism is impaired as a consequence of secondary nutrient deficiencies in iron and vitamins B_6 and B_{12}.[22]

To ensure optimal folate status, many countries have adopted folic acid fortification programs. The impetus for this political action spawned from the results of a series of trials conducted in the 1980s and 1990s, which demonstrated that maternal folic acid supplementation reduced the risk of giving birth to a baby with defects such as spina bifida.[23] Since its inception in 1998, folic acid fortification has resulted in an increase in folate concentrations and appears to decrease risk of neural tube defects[24] and cardiovascular disease[25] without increasing the number of elderly with low vitamin B_{12} status without anemia.[26] This is of concern, as folic acid supplementation may mask signs of vitamin B_{12} deficiency such as megaloblastic anemia. For this reason, the Dutch government has refrained from fortification of food products with folic acid meant for the general population.[27] Monitoring for adverse effects of folic acid is also necessary: maternal folic acid supplementation may increase risk of spontaneous abortion[28,29] and may increase the number of babies born with the 5,10-methylenetetrahydrofolate reductase (MTHFR) 677TT genotype.[30] Adverse effects of folic acid on risk of cancer are unknown.[31]

Functions of folate

Folate is essential for many physiological functions. Recent evidence suggests an antioxidant-like function of folate, but the traditional function of folate is that it accepts and donates one-carbon units (Figure 1.1). Various folate derivatives fulfill roles for one-carbon transfer for *de novo* nucleotide and formate synthesis and amino acid interconversions. The bulk of research on folate is attributed to its role with homocysteine, an amino acid formed in cells when the essential amino acid, methionine, is catabolized.[4] An elevated concentration of plasma total homocysteine is an independent risk factor for vascular disease.[32] Folic acid supplementation and extra dietary folate intake from the food may decrease concentrations of plasma homocysteine. Effect of low folate concentrations or folic acid supplementation on coenzyme Q_{10} has received less research.

Scientific optimism

But will folic acid prevent disease? There is much optimism for folate as a panacea. Governments hesitant with folic acid fortification have even been accused of public health malpractice.[33] Reviews have summarized the wealth of literature from *in vitro*, *in vivo*, animal and human studies, which have shown adverse changes in vascular and neurological tissue associated with low concentrations of folate and elevated concentrations of homocysteine. Likewise, observational studies have shown an independent association of folate and homocysteine with cardiovascular disease. A recent meta-analysis has found that a 2.6 μmol/L higher homocysteine was associated with a 13% (95% CI 8 to 19%) increase in risk of cardiovascular disease.[32] Cohort and case-cohort studies suggest that low folate intake[34-37] and low levels of serum or erythrocyte

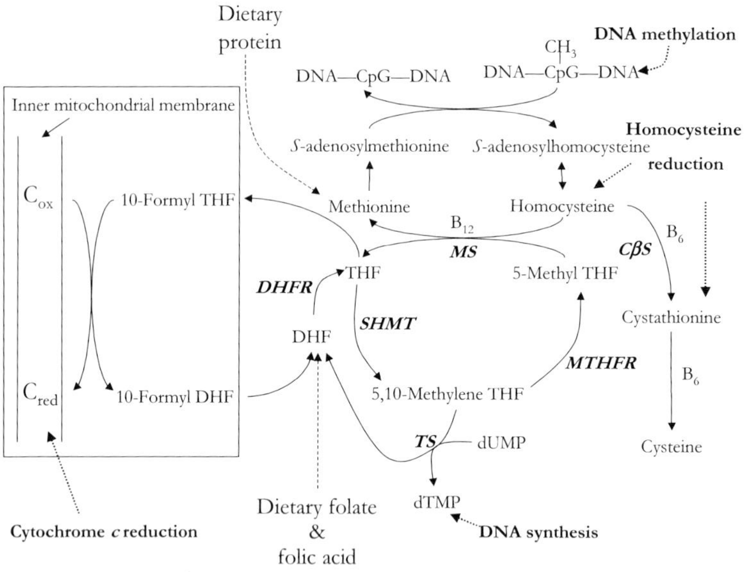

Figure 1.1 Metabolism and function of folate.
The MTHFR 677C→T polymorphism, involving a C to T substitution at the 677 base of the gene encoding for MTHFR, is associated with reduced enzyme activity *in vitro*. Subjects with the MTHFR 677TT genotype have in theory a reduced capacity of methyl transfer and greater capacity of formyl folate for i.e. mitochondrial cytochrome *c* reduction (mitochondria are the greatest producers of reactive oxygen species in the cell) and methenyl folate for thymidylate synthase, preventing dUMP accumulation, which has been associated with increased uracil misincorporation in DNA. Alongside the MTHFR 677TT genotype, low intracellular concentrations of folate can influence competition for 5,10-methylene-tetrahydrofolate, which favors commitment of one-carbon moieties for formylfolate and methenylfolate reactions.[46] Subjects with the MTHFR 677TT genotype have increased risk of cardiovascular disease and decreased risk of cancer. The association of the MTHFR 677TT genotype with dementia and neural tube defects is unclear. Abbreviations. DNA—CpG—DNA DNA CpG island; THF tetrahydrofolate; DHF dihydrofolate; MS methionine synthase; CβS cystathionine β-synthase; DHFR dihydrofolate reductase; SHMT serine hydroxymethyltransferase; MTHFR methylenetetrahydrofolate reductase; TS thymidylate synthase; dUMP deoxyuridylate; dTMP thymidylate; C_{ox} oxidized cytochrome *c*; C_{red} reduced cytochrome *c*.

folate,[36-45] independent of homocysteine concentrations,[37-39] are associated with vascular disease morbidity and mortality.

Some believe the evidence on the benefit for homocysteine-lowering by B vitamins is so strong that ethical issues have arisen in B vitamin trials. For example, patients enrolled in a B vitamin trial in the control group were not offered placebo, rather low-doses of B vitamins.[47] Alternatively, subjects with high homocysteine concentrations were excluded from folate trials as it was deemed unethical to allocate them to the placebo treatment (FACIT[1] trial).[48] A combination pill of 0.8 mg folic acid plus a statin, three antihypertensive agents and aspirin has been brought forth as a therapeutic strategy capable of reducing risk of stroke by 80% and risk of ischemic heart disease by 88% in individuals above 55 years of age.[49] In the case of folic acid, this risk reduction was based solely on observational evidence.[50] Some governments have endorsed health claims for folate. The USA, for example, has authorized the 'qualified health claim' for folic acid, vitamin B_{12} and vitamin B_6. "As part of a well-balanced diet, rich in fresh fruits and vegetables, daily intake of at least 400 μg folic acid, 3 mg vitamin B_6 and 5 μg vitamin B_{12} may reduce the risk of vascular disease."[51] Food manufacturers have put forth health claims suggesting benefit of extra folate (in their product) for the 'heart and mind.'

There is surprisingly little evidence from randomized controlled trials to support the B vitamin health claims for the reduction of vascular disease risk, let alone for improving cognitive function (Table 1.1). One study found a beneficial effect of B vitamin supplementation on restenosis after percutaneous transluminal coronary angioplasty after two years; this effect was confined to those subjects responsive to therapy as measured by homocysteine reduction (n=553).[52] In contrast, in a larger study, percutaneous transluminal coronary angioplasty patients administered B vitamin therapy, initially intravenously and thereafter orally, had smaller lumen diameters and increased rates of restenosis compared with patients taking the placebo (n=636).[53] Three studies found a positive effect of B vitamin supplementation on cardiovascular disease risk as measured by carotid intima-media thickness and abnormal exercise electrocardiography test.[54-56] The former is a validated surrogate marker of vascular disease[57] whereas the latter may be inappropriate as marker for cardiovascular disease risk in the general population.[58]

Limitations in evidence

Evidence for the health claims has not come from the trials, with ~8,000 subjects showing no effect of folic acid on cardiovascular disease risk, but has been based on evidence from observational epidemiology.[51] Observational epidemiology suffers from confounding and reverse causality. Confounding, because people with high folate levels differ in many aspects from those with lower levels. These aspects may be difficult to

[1] FACIT is an acronym for Folic Acid and Carotid Intima-media Thickness. The FACIT trial investigates the effects of 0.8 mg folic acid supplementation for three years on carotid intima-media thickness, cognitive function and hearing.

Table 1.1 Summary of studies investigating the effect of folic acid on vascular disease endpoints.[a]

Design	Duration	Sample size (*n*)	and Treatment	Relative risk (95% confidence interval)
Vascular disease				
RCT[59]	2 y	942	5 mg FA	1.0 (0.7 to 1.3) Revascularization, recurrent myocardial infarction, cardiac-cause death
		940	placebo	
RCT[47]	2 y	1827	2.5 mg FA, 25 mg B_6, 0.4 mg B_{12}	1.0 (0.8 to 1.1) Recurrent stroke
		1853	0.02 mg FA, 0.2 mg B_6, 6 μg B_{12}	
T[60]	20 m[b]	79	5 mg FA, 250 mg B_6[c]	0.96 (0.6 to 1.6) Recurrent peripheral disease, coronary or cerebrovascular disease
		194	standard care[d]	
T[61]	57 m[b]	52	5 mg FA, 250 mg B_6[c]	1.03 (0.6 to 1.9) Recurrent cerebrovascular disease, coronary or peripheral disease
		151	standard care[d]	
RCT[e]	6 m	353	5 mg FA, 50 mg B_6, 0.4 mg B_{12}	0.8 (0.6 to 1.3) Recurrent venous thrombosis
		348	placebo	
T[62,63]	5 y[b,f]	101	2.5 mg FA, 25 mg B_6, 0.25 mg B_{12}	-0.2 cm^2/y change in rate of carotid plaque progression
RCT[53]	6 m	316	1.2 mg FA, 48 mg B_6, 0.06 mg B_{12}[g]	1.5 (1.0 to 2.3) Revascularization target vessel, myocardial infarction, cardiac-cause death
		320	placebo	
RT[64]	1 y	140	5 mg FA, statin	0.98 (0.7 to 1.4) Recurrent myocardial infarction, stroke, invasive vascular intervention, all-cause death
		143	statin	
RT[65]	2 y[b]	300	0.5 mg FA	1.1 (0.6 to 1.8) Recurrent myocardial infarction, stroke, invasive vascular intervention, all-cause death
		293	standard care	
RCT[52]	6 m	272	1 mg FA, 10 mg B_6, 0.4 mg B_{12}	0.5 (0.3 to 0.9) Restenosis
		281	placebo	
RCT[66]	6 m	58	1 mg FA, 10 mg B_6, 0.4 mg B_{12}	0.3 (0.2 to 0.7) Restenosis
		55	placebo	
RCT[67]	1 y	272	1 mg FA, 10 mg B_6, 0.4 mg B_{12}	0.7 (0.5 to 0.96) Revascularization, myocardial infarction, all-cause death
		281	placebo (6 m treatment only)	
RCT[54]	1 y	50	2.5 mg FA, 25 mg B_6, 0.5 mg B_{12} or placebo	-0.15 mm in carotid intima-media thickness
Renal patients				
RCT[55]	6 m	25	5 mg FA, 50 mg B_6, 0.4 mg B_{12}	55% regression in carotid intima-media thickness
		28	placebo	
RT[68]	2 y	174	15 mg FA	1.6 (0.6 to 1.9) Cardiovascular events, death (15 mg FA vs. 1 mg FA)
		177	5 mg FA	0.9 (0.2 to 4.2) Cardiovascular events, death (5 mg FA vs. 1 mg. FA)
		177	1 mg FA	
General population				
RCT[56]	2 y	78	5 mg FA, 250 mg B_6	0.9 (0.6 to 1.3) Ankle brachial index
		80	placebo	1.0 (0.3 to 4.1) Peripheral stenosis
				0.9 (0.5 to 1.6) Carotid stenosis
				0.4 (0.2 to 0.9) Abnormal exercise ECG
RCT[69]	13 m[b]	68	5 mg FA, 250 mg B_6	0.5 (0.2 to 1.4) Abnormal magnetic resonance angiography
		73	placebo	

[a] Abbreviations. R randomized; C controlled; T trial; FA folic acid; ECG electrocardiography.
[b] Follow up time.
[c] Hyperhomocysteinemic.

[d] Non-hyperhomocysteinemic.
[e] M den Heijer. Personal communication.
[f] Follow up time before treatment 2.7 - 4.5 y, follow up time after treatment 1.6 - 1.8 y.
[g] First day treatment 1 mg FA, 5 mg B_6, 1 mg B_{12} intravenously.

measure and may highly correlate with folate, hindering statistical adjustment.[70] Diets high in folate tend to be high in other nutrients and macromolecules such as antioxidants and other vitamins, minerals, mono- and polyunsaturated fatty acids, n-3 fatty acids, fiber, phytochemicals and plant protein, which could explain its inverse association with risk of cardiovascular disease. Subjects with low folate and high homocysteine concentrations tend to have poor dietary patterns, which have been associated with risk of cardiovascular disease, and more unhealthy lifestyle risk factors, e.g. smoking and low physical activity.[11,12,16,17,71-73] Secondly, associations from observational epidemiology may be explained by reverse causality. Stronger associations of homocysteine with risk of cardiovascular disease are found from case-control (prone to bias by existing disease influencing homocysteine) rather than from cohort studies[74] and the association from cohort studies is stronger in patient populations than the in the general population.[75] This suggests that homocysteine may be a marker of vascular damage.

Mendelian randomization

Genetics, specifically common polymorphisms of folate-dependent enzymes, may give insight into the temporal relationship and better understand etiology of disease. Mendelian randomization, the random assortment of e.g. MTHFR 677T alleles to offspring, reduces bias and confounding, as exposure (genotype) is not likely to influence other risk factors. An association found between MTHFR 677T allele and disease may support the causal relation of folate or homocysteine with disease.[76] Moreover, Mendelian randomization reduces imprecision; genotype is more representative of 'usual' homocysteine concentrations than a one-off homocysteine measurement with its inherent measurement error.[77] An ideal polymorphism for Mendelian randomization is one that results in appreciable inter-genotype variation in serum markers, like that of a 25% increase in homocysteine concentrations in subjects with the 5,10-methylentetrahydrofolate reductase (MTHFR) 677TT genotype compared with the CC genotype (Figure 1.1).[78] If indeed folate or homocysteine is causally associated with risk, then support for such a role comes from the 16% (95% CI 5 to 28%) greater risk of coronary heart disease in ~30,000 patients with the MTHFR TT genotype compared with CC genotype.[78,79] This estimate is largely unconfounded and establishes a temporal relationship between homocysteine and cardiovascular disease. Genetic association studies, as illustrated by Klerk et al,[78] require large sample sizes to avoid spurious results and assumes that MTHFR is not a pleiotrophic gene.[80]

Health claims

Neither observational nor genetic studies can tell us whether folic acid supplementation will lead to a reduction in vascular disease. Health claims for folate need to be based on convincing evidence from randomized controlled trials to generate and maintain consumer confidence. To date the majority of trials have been conducted in patients with vascular disease; however, evidence must also come from trials conducted in the general population, if only because the vast majority of consumers are not patients. Such a trial would require a large study population and have a lengthy duration to collect enough cases with incident cardiovascular disease. Validated surrogate markers of disease for the general population are needed to make such trials feasible.

Trials will make or break the enthusiasm around folate, just like antioxidant vitamin trials did in the 1990s. Supplementation with β-carotene increased incidence of cardiovascular disease, especially pronounced in smokers,[81] a surprise for the research community considering that in observational epidemiology and *in vitro* studies, β-carotene was inversely associated with risk of cardiovascular disease. The lessons from the β-carotene trials have taught us that complex diet rather than single nutrient may be important.[82] The beneficial actions of nutrients from our diet may be the result of food synergy, which reflects the interplay between a prudent dietary pattern, food groups like whole grains, fruits and vegetables and vegetable constituents.[82] Randomized controlled trials show that food-base interventions can decrease risk of cardiovascular disease.[83] Whether strategies that increase consumption of folate-rich foods rather than relying on folic acid supplementation are more successful in effectively preventing cardiovascular disease remains to been seen. Like Marie Antoinette's solution to the hungry women who stormed the Palace of Versailles in Paris of 1789, "let them eat cake," foods fortified with folic acid may prove to be just as frivolous.

This thesis

Low concentrations of folate and high concentrations of homocysteine have been associated with a variety of diseases. Since health claims suggest beneficial effects of folate and extra folic acid on e.g. vascular disease, we need support from trials in the general population. The FACIT trial is a three-year double blind randomized controlled trial investigating effect of daily folic acid supplementation (0.8 mg/d) on cardiovascular disease risk in men and postmenopausal women aged 50 to 70 years. Our primary outcome is carotid intima-media thickness, a validated marker of cardiovascular risk in the general population.[57] Such a trial should be a prerequisite for and may help support or refute health claims that suppose that extra folic acid will indeed reduce the risk of vascular disease.

Secondary measures in the FACIT trial include arterial stiffness and parameters of vitality such as cognitive performance and hearing. Arterial stiffness has been associated with age-related arterial changes, atherosclerosis and vascular disease risk,[57] and increases in response to increased homocysteine concentrations after a methionine load.[84] The association of homocysteine with markers of arterial stiffness has been inconsistent.[85-88] Two trials in the general population[89,90] and one trial in patients with end-stage renal disease have not found a beneficial effect of B vitamin therapy on markers of arterial stiffness.[91] There is a wealth of literature from observational epidemiology that has shown an association of low folate and high homocysteine concentrations with poor cognitive performance.[92,93] Evidence from folate trials on cognitive function in the population is still inconclusive.[94] Many trials employed small study populations, lacked a control group or placebo treatment, allocated multiple interventions such that the effect of folate cannot be delineated or employed insensitive tests, like the Mini-Mental Screening Examination.[47,95-100] The FACIT trial has employed sensitive cognitive tests that are known to vary with age.[101] Finally, although age-related hearing loss is one of the most prevalent chronic conditions affecting the elderly, there has been little research on the link with nutrition. Low concentrations of folate have been inversely associated with hearing levels in some populations with age-related hearing loss,[102,103] however, no trials have been conducted to determine whether an increase in folate concentrations is associated with improvement in hearing thresholds.

The mechanisms, which may explain the association of low folate or high homocysteine with age-related conditions and disease, remain elusive. Oxidative stress is believed to play a role in endothelial dysfunction and subsequent inflammatory response.[104] However, B vitamin supplementation does not affect markers of oxidative stress as found in randomized controlled trials.[105-107] Although folic acid supplementation improves endothelial function as measured by flow-mediated dilation,[108] we have shown that one-year folic acid supplementation does not affect markers of endothelial dysfunction such as von Willebrand factor and tissue factor or markers of hemostasis.[109]

Finally, trials conducted in the general population have not been able to show beneficial effects of B vitamin supplementation on markers of inflammation such as vascular adhesion molecule-1 and C-reactive protein.[109,110]

In this thesis we present the relationship between low folate and high homocysteine concentrations, on the one hand, and risk of vascular disease, cognitive performance and hearing, on the other hand, using the baseline data of the FACIT trial. The *second chapter* provides an overview of the studies that have examined the association of folate and homocysteine with cardiovascular disease risk as measured by carotid intima-media thickness. The *third chapter* illustrates the association of folate and homocysteine with carotid intima-media thickness and carotid distension, a marker of arterial stiffness. The *fourth* and *fifth chapters* present the association of low folate and high homocysteine with cognitive performance and hearing, respectively. The *sixth chapter* is based on data collected after one-year intervention. There we examined whether one-year folic acid supplementation offers anti-inflammatory effects as measured by soluble intracellular adhesion molecule-1, oxidized low-density lipoprotein (LDL), autoantibodies against oxidized LDL and C-reactive protein. In the *seventh chapter*, the final chapter, we consider the role of folate and homocysteine in cardiovascular disease, cognitive decline and age-related hearing loss based on our findings. Suggestions for future research are also discussed. The FACIT trial researchers will report their findings in 2005 on the effect of three-year folic acid supplementation on cardiovascular disease risk, cognitive decline and age-related hearing loss.

Chapter 2

Homocysteine and carotid intima-media thickness: a critical appraisal of the evidence

Jane Durga, Petra Verhoef, Michiel L. Bots, Evert G. Schouten

Division of Human Nutrition, Wageningen University, Wageningen, The Netherlands
Wageningen Centre for Food Sciences, Wageningen, The Netherlands
Julius Center for Health Sciences and Primary Care, University Medical Center Utrecht, Utrecht, The Netherlands

Atherosclerosis 2004; 176: 1-19

Abstract

Aim This review examines the relationship between hyperhomocysteinemia, a risk factor for vascular disease, and carotid intima-media thickness, a valid marker of generalized atherosclerosis and future vascular disease risk. The relationship between two important determinants of hyperhomocysteinemia in the general population—folate status and the methylenetetrahydrofolate reductase (MTHFR) 677C→T polymorphism—and carotid intima-media thickness is also covered.

Methods We searched literature databases for articles examining homocysteine and carotid intima-media thickness published before September 2003.

Results We identified 54 studies. Observational studies generally failed to demonstrate a relationship between homocysteine and carotid intima-media thickness in homocystinuric, uremic, hypercholesterolemic or non-insulin dependent diabetes mellitus patients or in subjects with insulin insensitivity. Weak associations, but usually only in certain sub-populations were found in vascular disease patients and in population-based studies. B vitamins reduce the progression of carotid intima-media thickness in renal transplant recipients and vascular disease patients as demonstrated by two trials. The majority of studies demonstrated increased carotid intima-media thickness in individuals with the MTHFR 677TT genotype. Folate status showed no relation to carotid intima-media thickness.

Conclusion In non-patient populations, hyperhomocysteinemia is weakly associated with carotid intima-media thickness. The association of the 677C→T MTHFR polymorphism with CIMT further supports this finding. Lastly, folate levels may need to reach a critically low status before an association can be found between folate and carotid intima-media thickness. Larger trials in various population types are needed to determine whether folate alone or in combination with vitamins B_6 and B_{12} will slow down or even reverse atherosclerotic progression.

Introduction

Symptomatic vascular disease is preceded by atherosclerotic changes in the arterial system and is culminated by triggers such as plaque disruption and secondary thrombotic complications leading to vessel occlusion and subsequent ischemia. Clinical episodes manifest themselves, depending on the occlusion location, as ischemic heart disease, ischemic stroke or peripheral arterial disease. Mildly to severely elevated plasma concentrations of total homocysteine are positively associated with an increased risk of cerebral, coronary and peripheral vascular disease independent of traditional vascular disease risk factors.[32,111] However, hyperhomocysteinemia may merely be a marker of atherosclerotic renal dysfunction[112] or vascular damage.[113] Whether homocysteine exerts its effects via thrombotic or atherogenic mechanisms and whether it is involved in early or advanced stages of atherosclerosis is uncertain.

Homocysteine is located at the fork of two pathways in the metabolism of methionine, which relies on coenzymes derived from vitamin B_{12}, folate and vitamin B_6 (Figure 2.1). Excess homocysteine is released from the cell into the circulation and metabolized by

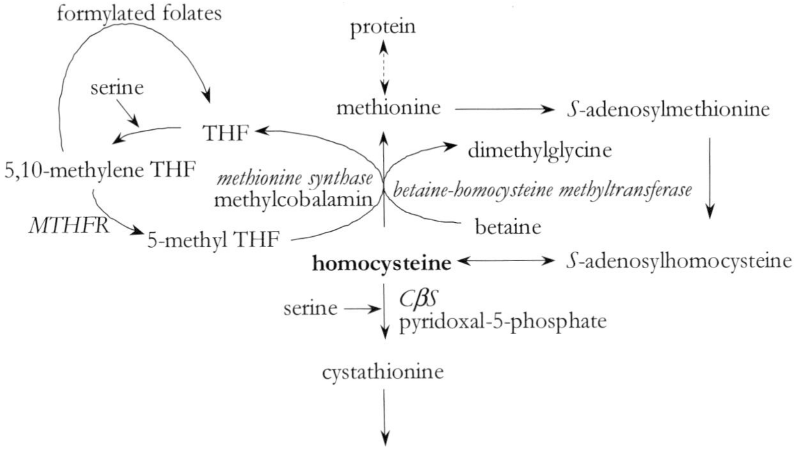

Figure 2.1 Homocysteine metabolism.
Homocysteine is the demethylated metabolite of methionine. The enzymes, MTHFR and methionine synthase, and the coenzymes, 5-methyltetrahydrofolate and methylcobalamin, are involved in homocysteine remethylation to form methionine. Irreversible transsulfuration of homocysteine to form cystathionine is dependent on cystathionine β-synthase and its coenzyme, pyridoxal-5-phosphate. Betaine-homocysteine methyltransferase can also remethylate homocysteine. The metabolic fate of homocysteine is dependent upon intracellular concentrations of *S*-adenosylmethionine, the primary methyl donor for physiological reactions. Abbreviations. MTHFR 5,10-methylenetetrahydrofolate reductase; THF tetrahydrofolate; CβS cystathionine β-synthase.

the liver and kidneys. Approximately two thirds of hyperhomocysteinemic cases are attributed to low B vitamin levels.[114] In addition, a 677C→T mutation in the gene encoding 5,10-methylenetetrahydrofolate reductase (MTHFR), a key enzyme in the remethylation cycle, increases homocysteine by approximately 25% in subjects with the MTHFR 677TT genotype. Supplementation with folic acid, vitamin B_{12} and vitamin B_6 can reduce homocysteine concentrations by approximately 33% in the general population.[115]

High resolution B-mode ultrasonography is a non-invasive method used to assess the combined thickness of the intimal and medial walls (Figure 2.2). Carotid intima-media thickness is a valid surrogate marker of vascular disease in the general and patient population: increased carotid intima-media thickness predicts vascular disease morbidity and mortality risk.[57] Furthermore, increased carotid intima-media thickness is a marker of atherosclerosis in other arterial beds.[117]

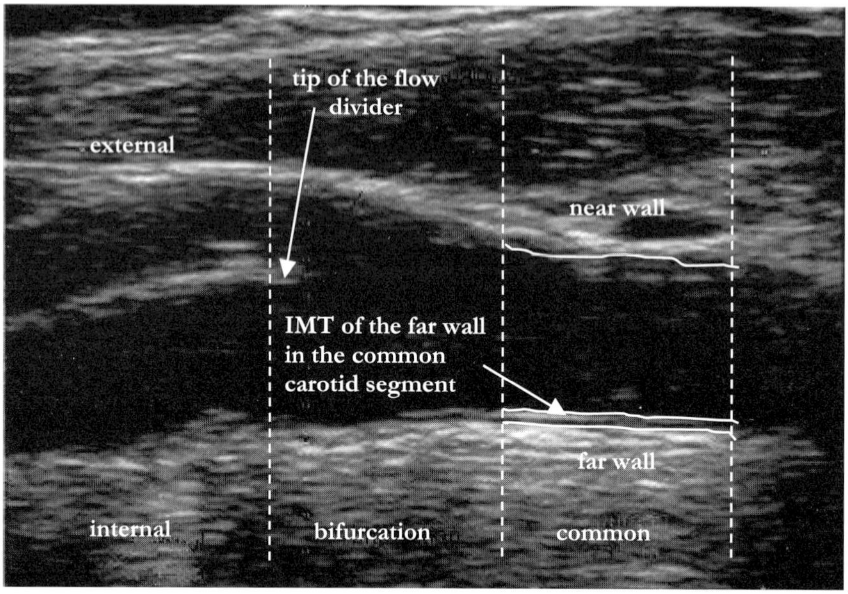

Figure 2.2 Distal common carotid artery.
The carotid artery is an elastic conduit artery that branches at the common to form the internal and external carotid arteries. Lesion progression and diffuse intimal-medial thickening in the carotid artery begins in the internal and the bifurcation and spreads proximally to the common carotid.[116] Carotid intima-media thickness methodologies vary according to the site, position and length of segment that is examined and to the computation using the far and/or near wall and segment length or point thickness. Carotid intima-media thickness estimates are reported as the mean or maximum thickness, as shown on this longitudinal ultrasound image.

This article systematically reviews the literature examining the relationship between homocysteine and carotid intima-media thickness in order to shed light on the role of homocysteine in vascular disease and atherogenesis, in particular. Special emphasis is given to folate status and the 677C→T MTHFR polymorphism, two important determinants of homocysteine in the general population.

Methods

English language literature published before September 2003 in Medline, Biological Abstracts and Current Contents databases were searched using "homocyst* and (carotid or thickness)" as key terms. All original studies conducted in humans were included if homocysteine and carotid intima-media thickness values were reported. In addition, references of articles found from the database search were scanned and experts in the homocysteine and carotid intima-media thickness fields were consulted for further suitable studies.

Results

Fifty-four articles were found. Five studies were excluded because data on the same population was presented.[118-122] Apart from two trials, the articles reported observational findings. Table 2.1 gives the main results of the studies whereas Figure 2.3 illustrates the mean homocysteine and carotid intima-media thickness per population subtype when reported by the authors. Carotid intima-media thickness is used in this article without reference to the segment measured; see Table 2.2 for the various carotid intima-media thickness protocols employed in each study.

Homocystinuria

McCully[123] brought forth the hypothesis that hyperhomocysteinemia is linked to vascular disease based on observations from patients with homozygous homocystinuria, an autosomal recessive condition characterized by hyperhomocysteinemia, hypermethioninemia and hypocysteinemia. Severe hyperhomocysteinemia (homocysteine >100 μmol/L) is caused by deficiency of the enzymes involved in methionine metabolism: cystathionine β-synthase, methionine synthase and MTHFR. Treatment regimens aimed at lowering homocysteine levels in homocystinuric patients appear to be protective against vascular disease,[124] although normalization of homocysteine is not always achieved.

Four cross-sectional studies examined homocysteine and carotid intima-media thickness in homocystinuric populations. The carotid intima-media thickness of heterozygous

Table 2.1 Summary of study characteristics and main outcome in relation to homocysteine and carotid intima-media thickness.[a]

Study Design[b]	Sample Size	Age (y) $\bar{x} \pm SD$	Inclusion Criteria	Homocysteine (μmol/L) $\bar{x} \pm SD$[c]	CIMT (mm) $\bar{x} \pm SD$[c]	Risk Association: Hcy and CIMT
Homocystinuria						
cross-sectional[125]	14 homozygote	13	CβS deficiency or remethylation errors	91 (range 9-179)	0.50 ± 0.01	Log Hcy β=0.025, adjusted for age and height in homozygotes and heterozygotes
	15 control	13	control: healthy, age matched	not measured	0.44 ± 0.01	
	15 heterozygote	41		14 (range 4-56)	0.50 ± 0.01	
	15 control	41		not measured	0.48 ± 0.01	
cross-sectional[86]	19 homozygote	44 ± 18	CβS deficiency, no DM, no renal dysfunction, no antihypertensive medication[d]	62.5 ± 43.6[e]	0.71 ± 0.14[e]	NG for homocystinuria, however in total population Hcy is not independent risk factor for CIMT
	14 heterozygote	36 ± 13		11.2 ± 1.3[e]	0.81 ± 0.19[e]	
	28 control	39 ± 11		10.6 ± 1.8[e]	0.70 ± 0.09[e]	
cross-sectional[126]	13 homozygote	33	CβS deficiency, <50 y	NG	0.59 ± 0.13	NG
	12 control	NG			0.59 ± 0.11	
cross-sectional[127]	25 heterozygote	42	CβS deficiency, <55 y	56 ± 28	NG	No significant difference in CIMT between groups
	21 control	NG	control: recruited from health screening	16 ± 5		
Uremia						
cross-sectional[149]	26 RTR	27 ± 6	childhood-onset chronic renal failure	23.5 ± 9.4	0.61 ± 0.11	Hcy not independent risk factor in uremics
	13 dialysis	27 ± 5		26 ± 10.6	0.66 ± 0.12	
	39 control	28 ± 6	control: healthy; age, sex, BMI, smoking	13.8 ± 3.5	0.54 ± 0.08	
cross-sectional[150]	129 ESRD	54 ± 15	ESRD: dialysis	29.2 ± 20.0	0.70 ± 0.15[f]	Hcy not independent risk factor for mean or max CIMT
	82 control	58 ± 13	control: non-uremic, CVD risk factor screening attendee or echocardiography patient	12.9 ± 4.9	0.61 ± 0.10[f]	
cross-sectional[151]	151 ESRD	55 ± 14	ESRD: dialysis, serum albumin <0.02 g/L[d]	23.1 ± 7.4	NG	Hcy not independent risk factor for CIMT in ESRD
	135 control	56 ± 12	control: healthy; age, sex matched	10.1 ± 5.0	not measured	
cross-sectional[152]	85	62 ± 14	dialysis, no carotid plaque	NG	0.67 ± 0.25	Hcy correlated with CIMT, no multivariate regression done
cross-sectional[153]	226	55 ± 14	dialysis, no CVD or cerebrovascular disease, no current infection 6 m prior to study	44.6 ± 19.1	0.92 ± 0.17 ♂ 0.87 ± 0.16 ♀	Hcy not independent risk factor for CIMT
cross-sectional[154]	55 ESRD	53 ± 12	ESRD: dialysis[g]	39.1 ± 27.2	0.74 ± 0.19	NG
	102 control	53 ± 7	hospital control: healthy, age, sex matched[g]	8.8 ± 2.7	0.66 ± 0.16	
cross-sectional[155]	33 RTR	43 ± 11	RTR	20.5 ± 5	0.68[h]	Hcy not independent risk factor for CIMT
	19 control	40 ± 7	population control	11.4 ± 6	0.54[h]	

cohort 1 y follow up[133]	53	NG	RTR, no DM, no CVD, no hypertension	NG	NG	Post-transplant: decline in Hcy, not related to CIMT regression
RCT 6 m[55]	25 active 28 placebo	49 ± 10 48 ± 10	RTR 1 y after transplant, no myocardial infarction or stroke, Hcy >15.5 µmol/L ♂ or >12.5 µmol/L ♀, no smoking, creatinine ≤133 µmol/L, creatinine decrease <15% in last 6 m[g] double blind: 5 mg folic acid, 50 mg B_6, 0.4 mg B_{12} or placebo	6 m 9.3 (5.8-13.0) 20.7 (15-34)	 0.64 ± 0.17 0.87 ± 0.19	B vitamin supplementation was associated with a 32 ± 13% decrease in CIMT, whereas in the placebo group, CIMT increased 23 ± 21% within 6 m
cross-sectional[156]	159 uremic 159 control	64 ± 8 NG	uremic: dialysis or creatinine >400 µmol/L population control: age, sex, smoking matched	27.7 ± 11.3 <13	0.89 ± 0.17 0.73 ± 0.13	Hcy no independent risk factor for CIMT
cross-sectional[157]	59	52	ESRD	25.1 ± 14.5	0.8 ± 0.3	Hcy correlated with CIMT (r=0.68, $p<0.001$), however, not significant after adjustment
cross-sectional[143]	60 ESRD 34 control	54 ± 14 50 ± 10	ESRD: dialysis, no DM, no CVD control: non-uremic; age, sex, blood pressure matched	36 ± 14 8.8 ± 1.2	0.79 ± 0.10 0.74 ± 0.10	Hcy not independent risk factor for CIMT
cross-sectional[148]	168 uremic 28 control	60 ± 14 61 ± 10	uremic: dialysis, no diabetic nephropathy[g] control: healthy	33.0 ± 16.9 11.0 ± 3.1	1.79 ± 1.16 NG	Hcy independent risk factor for CIMT in uremic patients (log Hcy β=0.198)
Cholesterolemia						
cross-sectional[158]	68 case 194 control	56 ± 11 48 ± 12	case: FH, vascular disease onset <55 y control: FH, no vascular disease	11.1 ± 4.9 10.1 ± 3.8	0.74 ± 0.16 0.69 ± 0.15	NG
cross-sectional[159]	22 homozygote 20 heterozygote 20 control	24 ± 10 32 ± 12 31 ± 4	FH, no smoking, no hypertension, no DM control: normocholesterolemic, no family history of CAD	7.3 ± 2.1 8.7 ± 4.4 9.3 ± 3.3	1.45 ± 0.4 0.76 ± 0.1 0.65 ± 0.7	Hcy not correlated to CIMT
cross-sectional[86]	21 homozygote 28 control	46 ± 11 39 ± 11	FH, no DM, no renal dysfunction, no antihypertensive medication	9.6 ± 1.4 10.6 ± 1.8	0.98 ± 0.29[e] 0.70 ± 0.09[e]	NG for FH, however in total population Hcy is not independent risk factor for CIMT
cross-sectional[160]	90 homozygote 30 control	NG 14 ± 2	FH, no smoking, age 10-19 y	6[h] 6[h]	0.48 ± 0.07[e] 0.46 ± 0.06[e]	Hcy independent risk factor for CCA and BIF
cross-sectional[161]	513	NG	total cholesterol ≥5 mmol/L, no uncontrolled hypertension, age 45-69 y	10.6 ± 2.8 ♂ 9.4 ± 2.3 ♀	1.05 ± 0.35 ♂ 0.89 ± 0.26 ♀	0.10 mm CIMT difference (≥11.5 µmol/L vs. <11.5 µmol/L) in ♂; adjusted for age, BMI
Diabetes						
cross-sectional[162]	124	65 ± 8	NIDDM, no ESRD	11.3 ± 5.1	0.9 ± 0.3	Hcy not independent risk factor for CIMT
cross-sectional[163]	130	53 ± 10	NIDDM, no renal disease, no CVD	7.8 ± 2.1	0.86 ± 0.22	Hcy not independent risk factor for CIMT
cross-sectional[164]	103	58	58 y, ♂, no CVD, no CVD medication[i]	13.0 ± 2.9	0.80 ± 0.12	Hcy not independent risk factor for CIMT
cross-sectional[165]	140 cases 91 controls	67 ± 7 71 ± 6	DM or impaired glucose intolerance, population-based	10.2 (8.4-12.5) 11.0 (9.6-13.8)	0.86 ± 0.2 0.88 ± 0.2	Hcy independent risk factor for CIMT (β=0.070)

Table 2.1 (*Continued*).

Study Design[b]	Sample Size	Age (y) $\bar{x} \pm$ SD	Inclusion Criteria	Homocysteine (µmol/L) $\bar{x} \pm$ SD[c]	CIMT (mm) $\bar{x} \pm$ SD[c]	Risk Association: Hcy and CIMT
Immune disorders						
cross-sectional[166]	423	41± 9	HIV clinic attendee, HIV-1 infection	12.3 ± 4.7	0.54 (0.50-0.60)	Hcy not independent risk factor for CIMT
cross-sectional[167]	42	31 ± 10	idiopathic antiphospholipid antibodies	13 ± 1.8	CCA 0.44 ± 0.01 ICA 0.41 ± 0.01 BIF 0.48 ± 0.02	Hcy independent risk factor for ICA (β=0.405) and BIF (β=0.404), but not CCA CIMT
cross-sectional[168]	26 SLE w/ CVD 26 SLE w/o CVD 26 control	52 ± 8 52 ± 8 52 ± 8	SLE w/ CVD: SLE, CVD, ♀ SLE w/o CVD: SLE, no CVD, ♀ population control: no SLE, no CVD, ♀	19.2 ± 9.6 15.0 ± 5.1 11.6 ± 3.8	0.66 ± 0.15 0.60 ± 0.14 0.59 ± 0.12	NG
Parkinson's disease						
cross-sectional[169]	100 case 100 control	72 ± 9	Parkinson's disease, no drug-induced or vascular Parkinsonism, no VD history	NG	0.88 ± 0.24 0.75 ± 0.18	Hcy not independent risk factor for CIMT
Suspected or confirmed vascular disease						
cross-sectional[170]	45 stenosis 20 occlusion 35 control	48 ± 4 48 ± 5 48 ± 6	stenosis: ≥30% stenosis of ICA, <55 y occlusion: ≥30% occlusion of ICA, <55 y hospital control: no plaque or stenosis in carotids, age, sex matched All subjects are neurological patients	11.7 ± 5.7 15.3 ± 8.4 10.4 ± 2.9	1.1 (0.71-1.63)[h] 1.0 (0.70-1.56)[h] 0.82 (0.64-1.26)[h]	Hcy not independent risk factor for CIMT in total population
cross-sectional[171]	120	77 ± 9	in-patients, ≥60 y	NG	NG	OR 3 vs. 1 tertile 6.49 (CI, 1.95 to 21.9); adjusted for age, sex, BMI, smoking, hypertension, DM, total cholesterol, triglycerides, HDL, creatinine; increased CIMT not defined
cross-sectional[172]	1467	56 ± 11	siblings of patients with CVD events, >25 y	9.5 ± 5.0	0.81 ± 0.29	4 and 5 vs. 1, 2 and 3 quintiles have significantly greater CIMT in ≥ 55 y only
case-control[173]	91 case 100 control	64 ± 10 52 ± 15	case: CIMT >2 mm of FW or NW of BIF or ICA, high risk out-patients control: CIMT<1.2 mm, high risk out-patients No methotrexate use, no renal disease[g]	11.7 ± 6.5 8.1 ± 4.4	NG	OR 1.11 (CI, 1.03 to 1.19); adjusted for age, sex, hypertension

RCT 12 m[54]	50	60 ± 8	patients, CIMT ≥1 mm double blind: 2.5 mg folic acid, 25 mg B_6, 0.5 mg B_{12} or placebo	12 m 6.6 ± 1.5 10.5 ± 3.3	Δ12 m -0.08 ± 0.17 0.07 ± 0.25	B vitamin supplementation for 6 m and 12 m was associated with a decrease in CIMT, CIMT increased in the placebo group
cross-sectional[174]	440	68 ± 4	CVD risk factor screening attendee, no CVD, ♂, creatinine <177 µmol/L, albumin ≥34 g/L	11.2 ± 4.1[j] 10.1 ± 3.1[k]	NG	OR 3 vs. 1 tertile 2.15 (CI, 1.11 to 4.16) for CIMT >1.0 mm CCA or >1.4 mm ICA; adjusted for age OR 3 vs. 1 tertile 5.80 (CI, 1.24 to 27.1) in non-hypertensives only; adjusted for age, DM, smoking, hypercholesterolemia
cross-sectional[175]	92	65 ± 9	patients referred for ECG, ≥50 y	11 ± 5	0.9 ± 0.2 CCA 1.2 ± 0.3 BIF	Hcy not independent risk factor for CIMT
cross-sectional[176]	144	NG	CVD risk factor screening attendee, CCA IMT ≤1 mm, no stenosis, no CVD, never user of antihypertensive medication	9.7 ± 2.8	Hcy tertiles 1st 0.51 ± 0.09 2nd 0.53 ± 0.09 3rd 0.54 ± 0.13	Hcy independent risk factor for CIMT (unstandardized β=0.0071)
cross-sectional[177]	10 normotensive 10 hypertensive 10 hypertensive w/ organ damage	50 ± 2 48 ± 3 50 ± 5	out-patients, 12-16 m post-menopausal ♀	5.4 ± 1.6 12.7 ± 3.4 24.3 ± 8.9	0.68 0.92 1.05	Hcy correlated with CIMT in hypertensives with and without organ damage (r=0.7 and r=0.5, respectively); Not stated whether correlation is adjusted for confounders
General population						
cross-sectional[178]	452 ♂ 659 ♀	64 ± 10 63 ± 10	>40 y	12.6 ± 5.5 9.8 ± 2.7	0.75 ± 0.22 0.67 ± 0.18	Hcy independent risk factor for CIMT (β=0.028)
cross-sectional[179]	1111	52 ± 13	no carotid surgery	12.1 ± 4.0	0.71 ± 0.14	OR 4 vs. 1 quartile 2.60 (CI, 1.51 to 4.45); adjusted for age, sex, systolic blood pressure, LDL, smoking, WHR, VaD and hypertension history, DM
case-control[180]	287 case 287 control	NG NG	case: ≥90th percentile of IMT of ARIC cohort control: ≤75th percentile of IMT of ARIC cohort no CVD, 45-64 y	9.3 8.3	1.21 0.63	Paired OR 1.78 (CI, NG) p>0.05 adjusted for HDL, age, WHR, smoking
cross-sectional[181]	630	68 ± 7	≥55 y	14.7 ± 4.3 <75 y 16.3 ± 4.3 ≥75 y	0.75 ± 0.13 <75 y 0.88 ± 0.17 ≥75 y	CIMT difference 0.037 mm (CI, 0.0004 to 0.074 mm) (Hcy ≥18.6 vs. <18.6 µmol/L) in <75 y only; adjusted for age and sex.
cross-sectional[182]	202 white 89 African Caribbean	64 ± 8 60 ± 8	♂, 40-75 y, white or African Caribbean descent	13.9 ± 4.9 14 ± 6.7	0.76 ± 0.01[f] 0.81 ± 0.01[f]	Hcy not independent risk factor for CIMT

Table 2.1 (*Continued*).

Study Design[b]	Sample Size	Age (y) $\bar{x} \pm SD$	Inclusion Criteria	Homocysteine (µmol/L) $\bar{x} \pm SD^c$	CIMT (mm) $\bar{x} \pm SD^c$	Risk Association: Hcy and CIMT
cross-sectional[85,l]	614 ♂ 595 ♀	60	NG	10.6[m] 8.5[m]	0.70 0.70	Hcy not independent risk factor for CIMT
cross-sectional[183,l]	819	NG	50-70 y	13.3 ± 2.9	mean 0.83 ± 0.13 max 1.02 ± 0.17	Hcy not independent risk factor for CIMT
cross-sectional[184]	1077	72 ± 7	60-90 y	11.5 ± 4.1	NG	Hcy not independent risk factor for CIMT
cross-sectional[185]	721 ♂ 820 ♀	60 ± 13 58 ± 12	30-89 y	13.3 ± 4.2[n] 10.7 ± 3.0[n]	mean 0.88 ± 0.14 max 1.15 ± 0.45[e] mean 0.83 ± 0.12 max 1.02 ± 0.29[e]	Partial correlation coefficient 0.15-0.36 for Hcy and maximum CIMT in ♂ only, depending on C677T MTHFR genotype; adjusted for age, BMI, drinking, smoking, systolic blood pressure, hypertension medication use, hyperlipidemia, DM. Hcy not associated with mean CIMT.
cross-sectional[186]	120	62 ± 4	normal glucose tolerance, normotensive, ♀, creatinine <106 µmol/L, total cholesterol <6.5 mmol/L, no CVD or HRT[g]	10.6 ± 2.4	1.23 ± 0.04 TT 1.03 ± 0.02 CT 0.98 ± 0.04 CC	Hcy independent risk factor for CIMT (β=0.286); CIMT continuous variable Hcy not independent risk factor for CIMT when using 1 mm cut-off
cross-sectional[187]	75	49 ± 16	normal creatinine and folate, no medication use, normotensive, no CVD	10.5 ± 2.8	0.78 ± 0.19	Partial R^2=0.1077, model R^2=0.367 After adjusted for age, BMI, LDL, systolic blood pressure; 18% of variation in CIMT was explained by Hcy

[a] Abbreviations. CIMT carotid intima-media thickness; SD standard deviation; CβS cystathionine β-synthase; DM diabetes mellitus; NG not given; RTR renal transplant recipients; BMI body mass index; ESRD end stage renal disease; CVD cardiovascular disease; RCT randomized controlled trial; FH familial hypercholesterolemia; CAD coronary artery disease; CCA common carotid artery; BIF carotid bifurcation; NIDDM non-insulin dependent diabetes mellitus; HIV-1 human immunodeficiency virus type 1; ICA internal carotid artery; SLE systemic lupus erythematosus; OR odds ratio; CI 95% confidence interval; LDL low-density lipoprotein cholesterol; WHR waist hip ratio; VaD vascular disease; ARIC Atherosclerosis Risk in Communities Study; HDL high-density lipoprotein cholesterol; FW far wall; NW near wall; ECG electrocardiography; max maximum; HRT hormone replacement therapy; ♂ men; ♀ women.

[b] Association of homocysteine with carotid intima-media thickness.

[c] Median (interquartile range).

[d] Received B vitamin supplements.

[e] Fasting homocysteine and/or CCA FW.

[f] Adjusted mean ± standard error.

[g] No folate or B vitamin supplementation.
[h] Approximate.
[i] Selection based on insulin sensitivity score.
[j] Hypertensives.
[k] Non-hypertensives.
[l] Data extracted from abstract.
[m] Geometric mean.
[n] Estimates based on larger study population.

homocystinurics was similar to healthy control,[86,125-127] even when heterozygotes had high concentrations of homocysteine compared with controls,[126,127] With one exception,[125] the presence of hyperhomocysteinemia in homozygous homocystinurics[86,125] was not paired with greater carotid intima-media thickness compared with controls.[86,128,129] Apart from the small sample sizes, heterogeneity in the populations explains the disparate results. The study that found a positive relation between homozygous homocystinuria and increased carotid intima-media thickness included younger participants with overt vascular disease and pyridoxine non-responsive participants (those responsive to pyridoxine treatment had normal carotid intima-media thickness) with remethylation metabolic errors rather than cystathionine β-synthase deficiency only.[125]

In summary, these results suggest that hyperhomocysteinemia is not associated with carotid intima-media thickness in homocystinurics. The nature of arteriosclerosis is unique in homocystinuria—intimal hyperplasia in the absence of lipid-laden atheromas and medial thinning—and has been suggested to explain similar carotid intima-media thickness found in homocystinurics compared with controls despite the presence of hyperhomocysteinemia.[129] Atypical arteriosclerosis may be explained by other disturbances associated with errors in the methionine metabolism. For example, cystathionine β-synthase deficiency-related hypocysteinemia is associated with diminished deposition of fibrillin-1, a major constituent of elastic microfibrils, in the extracellular matrix.[130]

Uremia

Prospective studies in uremic patients demonstrated an independent relation between homocysteine and cardiovascular disease morbidity and mortality.[131] It is possible that hyperhomocysteinemia due to renal impairment will accelerate atherosclerosis although some researchers contend that hyperhomocysteinemia is merely a marker of renal dysfunction. Indeed, homocysteine is sensitive to changes in renal function as measured by glomerular filtration rate, serum creatinine and creatinine clearance[132] or due to successful renal transplantation.[133] In addition to the importance of the kidneys in homo-

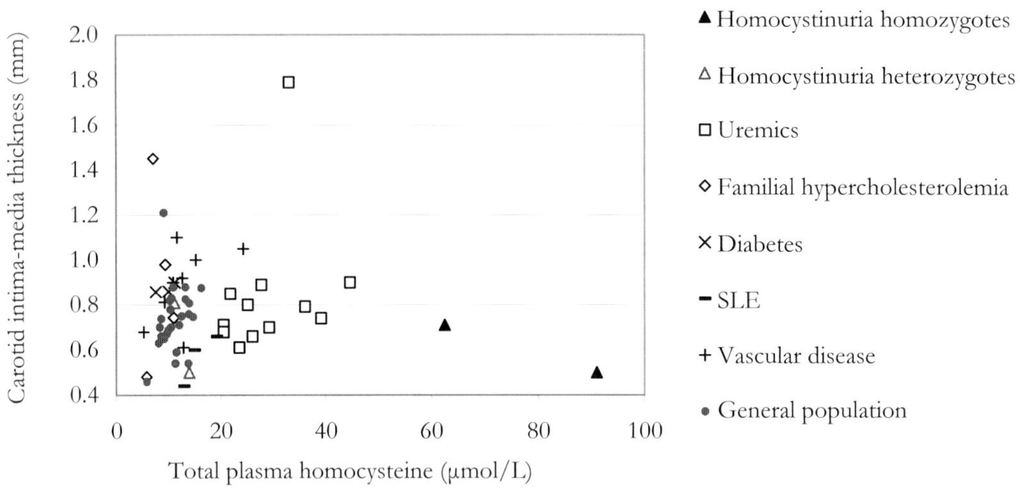

Figure 2.3 Scatter plot of homocysteine and carotid intima-media thickness.

An illustration of some of the populations described in this review, based on mean or median homocysteine and carotid intima-media thickness. The populations with the highest homocysteine values do not necessarily have the greatest carotid intima-media thickness, e.g. homocystinurics and uremic patients. Vice versa, those with the greatest carotid intima-media thickness do not necessarily have hyperhomocysteinemia, e.g. familial hyper-cholesterolemia. Abbreviations. SLE systemic lupus erythematosus.

homocysteine metabolism and clearance, decreased folate levels may lead to hyperhomocysteinemia. Loss of folate due to dialysis,[134] decreased transmembrane transport of folate[135] and/or decreased folate conjugase activity[136] help explain the often-suboptimal folate concentrations and subsequent hyperhomocysteinemia in uremic patients. Unfortunately, homocysteine is often intractable to treatments that enhance remethylation, i.e. folic acid, betaine or serine.[91,137,138] This suggests that hyperhomocysteinemia in uremia is to a great extent a reflection of extracellular accumulation because of renal dysfunction, rather than a perturbed intracellular remethylation process.

All studies that compared uremic patients to non-uremic controls confirmed that in uremic patients homocysteine concentrations[139-146] and carotid intima-media thickness[140-147] were greater; nevertheless, homocysteine was independently associated with carotid intima-media thickness in only one study.[148] This cross-sectional study excluded subjects taking B vitamin supplements so that homocysteine concentrations probably reflected the juxtaposition of two types of hyperhomocysteinemia: B vitamin intractable-hyperhomocysteinemia due to renal dysfunction and B vitamin responsive-hyperhomocysteinemia associated with perturbed remethylation processes. Carotid intima-media thickness measurements differed from other studies conducted in uremics: severity of atherosclerosis was estimated (i.e. the maximum thickness of any carotid segment). That homocysteine may be associated with severity rather than extent of atherosclerosis, is supported by a recent cross-sectional study in dialysis patients which illustrated that homocysteine was associated with carotid plaque score, but not with carotid intima-media thickness.[157]

Two observational studies examined the relation between homocysteine and carotid intima-media thickness in renal transplant recipients.[133,155] One case-control study demonstrated that renal transplant recipients had greater carotid intima-media thickness and homocysteine than healthy controls, however, homocysteine was not associated with carotid intima-media thickness.[155] The second study examined changes in homocysteine and carotid intima-media thickness in 53 patients every three months after renal transplantation. All patients attained normohomocysteinemic levels after one year. Despite the drastic reduction in homocysteine, no effect of renal transplantation on carotid intima-media thickness progression was detected in the group with initial homocysteine ≥40 µmol/L. Paradoxically, only patients with normal and moderate levels of homocysteine demonstrated a slight decrease in carotid intima-media thickness thickening.[133] Finally, a randomized double blind controlled trial showed beneficial effects of daily B vitamin supplementation (5 mg folic acid, 0.4 mg vitamin B_{12} and 50 mg vitamin B_6) in 56 stable renal transplant recipients with homocysteine concentrations ≥15.5 µmol/L and ≥12.5 µmol/L for men and women, respectively.[55] Baseline homocysteine and carotid intima-media thickness were approximately 20 µmol/L and 0.86±0.17 mm, respectively. After six months, in the B vitamin group homocysteine declined by 64±12% and carotid intima-media thickness regressed 32±13%, whereas in the placebo group homocysteine remained at 20 µmol/L and carotid intima-media thickness progressed 23±21%. The sudden change in carotid intima-media thickness was not accompanied by a decline in blood pressure nor total cholesterol.

In summary, from observation studies there is scarce evidence that homocysteine is related to carotid intima-media thickness in uremic patients, although few studies were designed to examine this issue specifically. The effects of renal dysfunction on atherosclerosis may overshadow any association of homocysteine with carotid intima-

Table 2.2 B-mode sonography methodology used in the reviewed studies.[a]

Carotid intima-media thickness	Segment and position[b]		FW & NW
Homocystinuria			
NG[125]	CCA[c]	NG	FW
mean[86]	CCA	distal 1 cm	FW & NW
	ICA	proximal 1 cm	FW
	BIF	NG	NG
mean[126]	CCA	distal	FW
	ICA	proximal	
	BIF	NG	
mean[127]	CCA	1 cm proximal to BIF	FW
Uremia			
maximum[149]	CCA[d]	2-4 cm proximal to BIF	FW
mean and maximum[150]	CCA	1 cm proximal to BIF, plaque-free	FW & NW
mean[151]	CCA	1 cm proximal to bulb dilatation	FW & NW
NG[152]	CCA	distal 1 cm CCA	NG
mean[153]	CCA	distal CCA	FW
mean[154]	CCA	1 cm proximal to bulb dilatation, plaque-free	FW
mean[155]	CCA	NG	FW
	BIF	NG	
mean of maximum[133]	CCA	NG	FW
NG[55]	CCA[d]	2-4 cm proximal to BIF	FW
mean[156]	CCA	distal CCA	NG
NG [157]	CCA	0.5-1 cm proximal to BIF	FW
NG[143]	CCA[e]	2 cm proximal to BIF	FW
maximum[148]	CCA	distal 1 cm	NW
	ICA	proximal 1 cm	
	BIF	NG	
Cholesterolemia			
NG[158]	NG[e]	NG	NG
NG[159]	CCA[e]	NG	FW
mean[86]	CCA	distal 1 cm	FW & NW
	ICA	proximal 1 cm	FW
	BIF	NG	NG
mean and maximum[160]	CCA[c]	distal 1 cm	FW
	BIF[c]	proximal 1 cm	
mean of maximum[161]	CCA	at site of maximum CIMT	FW
Diabetes			
mean[162]	CCA	site of max CIMT, 1 cm up and down from maximum	FW
mean[163]	CCA	1 cm proximal to bulb dilatation, plaque-free	FW
mean[164]	CCA	NG	FW
mean[165]	CCA[c]	1 cm proximal to bulb	FW
Immune disorders			
NG[166]	CCA[f]	distal	FW
mean[167]	CCA	distal 1 cm	FW
	ICA	distal 1 cm	
	BIF	distal 1 cm	

Table 2.2 (*Continued*).

Carotid intima-media thickness	Segment and position[b]		FW & NW
mean[168]	CCA	NG	FW
Parkinson's disease			
maximum[169]	CCA[e]	3 cm proximal to flow divider	FW & NW
	ICA[e]	distal 1.5 cm	
	ECA[e]	distal 1.5 cm	
	BIF[e]		
Suspected or confirmed vascular disease			
mean[170]	CCA	1 cm proximal to bulb dilatation	FW
mean[171]	CCA	1 cm proximal to BIF	FW
mean[172]	CCA	1 cm proximal to bulb dilatation	FW
	ICA	1 cm distal to flow divider	
	BIF	1 cm proximal to flow divider	
NG[173]	CCA	1 cm below BIF	FW & NW
	ICA	1 cm above BIF	
NG[54]	NG	NG	NG
maximum[174]	CCA	distal 1 cm	FW & NW
	ICA	beginning of dilatation until 1 cm distal to tip of flow divider	
mean and maximum[175]	CCA	distal 1 cm	FW
	BIF	NG	
NG[176]	CCA[c]	2 cm beneath BIF	FW
NG[177]	NG	NG	NG
General population			
mean[178]	CCA[e]	1-3 cm proximal to BIF	FW & NW
mean[179]	CCA	distal 1 cm, plaque-free	FW
mean[180]	CCA	NG	FW & NW
	ICA	NG	
	BIF	NG	
mean[181]	CCA	NG	FW & NW
mean and maximum[182]	CCA	2 cm proximal to flow divider	FW
mean[85,g]	NG[e]	NG	NG
mean and maximum[183,g]	CCA	distal	NG
NG[184]	NG	NG	NG
mean and maximum[185]	CCA	1 cm proximal to bulb dilation	FW & NW
mean of maximum[186]	CCA	1-2 cm proximal to bulb, upstream to eventual plaque	FW & NW
mean[187]	CCA[d]	1 cm proximal to BIF	FW

[a] Abbreviations. FW far wall; NW near wall; CCA common carotid artery; NG not given; ICA internal carotid artery; BIF carotid bifurcation; ECA external carotid artery.
[b] Right and left carotids.
[c] Right carotid only.
[d] Side with the greatest carotid intima-media thickness.
[e] No specification of carotid side.
[f] Left carotid only.
[g] Data extracted from abstract.

media thickness: renal dysfunction has been associated with a unique atherosclerotic pathobiology.[188] It is also plausible that hyperhomocysteinemia due to extracellular accumulation, in contrast with an intracellular remethylation imbalance, does not lead to atherosclerosis. The promising findings from a recent trial in hyperhomocysteinemic renal transplant recipients that B vitamins lead to carotid intima-media thickness regression, needs to be confirmed, also in other types of uremic populations.

Hypercholesterolemia

Individuals with familial hypercholesterolemia have an increased risk of intimal-medial thickening and vascular disease. In an environment of elevated low-density lipoprotein (LDL) cholesterol with enhanced interstitial LDL in the intima, it is feasible that hyperhomocysteinemia exacerbates the accelerated atherogenesis seen in hypercholesterolemic individuals. Familial hypercholesterolemia individuals have LDL cholesterol which is less susceptible to oxidation[189] and similar auto-antibodies titers to oxidized LDL as controls.[190] Furthermore, 8-isoprostanes, a product of LDL oxidative reactions, is not associated with carotid intima-media thickness in familial hypercholesterolemia patients.[159] Lastly, neither carotid intima-media thickness nor homocysteine is associated with the risk of premature heart disease in familial hypercholesterolemia patients.[158]

Four studies conducted in familial hypercholesterolemia populations measured homocysteine and carotid intima-media thickness.[86,158-160] Familial hypercholesterolemia patients had similar homocysteine to controls. Familial hypercholesterolemia homozygotes had increased carotid intima-media thickness compared with heterozygotes, and heterozygotes had a thicker intimal-medial wall complex than controls. LDL cholesterol was the unanimous predictor of carotid intima-media thickness across the studies; homocysteine was not associated with carotid intima-media thickness in these populations.[86,159] To determine whether hyperhomocysteinemia at an early age influences carotid intima-media thickness, one cross-sectional study was conducted in children with familial hypercholesterolemia.[160] Familial hyper-cholesterolemia children had similar homocysteine and carotid intima-media thickness to controls; however, homocysteine was an independent risk factor for carotid intima-media thickness.

A cross-sectional study conducted in hypercholesterolemic (≥5.0 mmol/L LDL cholesterol) men and postmenopausal women has shown that the mean adjusted carotid intima-media thickness was 0.10 mm greater in the upper homocysteine quartile compared with the lower quartiles in men only.[161] The population-based homocysteine quartiles used (rather than sex-based quartiles) led to a small group of women in the highest homocysteine quartile, compromising the power to test this interaction.

LDL cholesterol, and not homocysteine, predicts carotid intima-media thickness in familial hypercholesterolemia patients. One could speculate that prolonged exposure to hypercholesterolemia might overshadow a relation between homocysteine and carotid intima-media thickness, as has been demonstrated in animal studies.[191]

Diabetes

In diabetic patients, homocysteine is a more potent risk factor for all-cause mortality than in non-diabetics.[192] Resistance to postprandial lowering of homocysteine in non-insulin dependent diabetes mellitus patients[193] and increased advanced glycation end-product receptor concentration[194] may in part be responsible for increased susceptibility to vascular disease. Unless there is concurrent diabetic nephropathy, homocysteine tends to be lower in diabetics than in non-diabetics possibly due to glomerular hyperfiltration[195] or increased hepatic transsulfuration.[196]

Two studies in non-insulin dependent diabetes mellitus patients and one study in generally healthy men recruited based on insulin sensitivity have not been able to demonstrate a relation between homocysteine and carotid intima-media thickness, even when the analyses were confined to subjects with increased carotid intima-media thickness.[162-164] Recently, however, homocysteine was associated with carotid intima-media thickness in patients with non-insulin dependent diabetes mellitus or subjects with impaired glucose tolerance.[165] This association was independent of confounders and B vitamins. When the authors excluded subjects with known diabetes, the association of homocysteine with carotid intima-media thickness persisted.

Immune disorders

The major cause of morbidity and mortality in patients with systemic lupus erythematosus is vascular disease. Premature vascular disease is a consequence of the systemic lupus erythematosus disease process, i.e. premature atherosclerosis, vasculitis and hypercoagulability, and of systemic lupus erythematosus medications like corticosteroid and methotrexate treatment that increase homocysteine concentrations.[197] Hyperhomocysteinemia led to 3.5-fold increase in arterial thrombosis risk and a 2.4-fold increase in stroke risk after adjustment for vascular disease risk factors in systemic lupus erythematosus populations.[198]

One study investigated homocysteine in two systemic lupus erythematosus populations, those with and those without arterial disease, compared with population controls.[168] Homocysteine and carotid intima-media thickness were greater in systemic lupus erythematosus cases than in the systemic lupus erythematosus controls. Although homocysteine was significantly elevated in systemic lupus erythematosus controls, they did not have greater carotid intima-media thickness than the population controls; that systemic lupus erythematosus does not confer a greater carotid intima-media thickness is in agreement with a recent study.[199] In a second study, homocysteine was independently related to carotid intima-media thickness in the bifurcation and internal carotid artery, but not in the common carotid artery in patients with idiopathic antiphospholipid antibodies.[167] This condition commonly occurs in autoimmune disorders.

Finally, the use of a cocktail of protease and reverse transcriptase inhibitors to treat human immunodeficiency virus type 1 (HIV-1) has been associated with an atherogenic profile, including lipodystrophy syndrome, hyperlipidemia and insulin resistance. In HIV-1 infected patients, homocysteine was not related to carotid intima-media thickness after adjustment for conventional cardiovascular risk factors.[166]

Parkinson's disease

L-3,4-dihydroxyphenylalanine (L-DOPA), a drug used for Parkinson's disease therapy, is associated with hyperhomocysteinemia[200,201] and has been hypothesized to increase the risk of vascular disease in patients with Parkinson's disease.[169] The association of homocysteine with carotid intima-media thickness was examined in 100 Parkinson's disease patients treated with L-DOPA, however homocysteine was not associated with carotid intima-media thickness.[169]

Confirmed or suspected vascular disease patient population

The evidence for an association of hyperhomocysteinemia with increased risk of vascular disease is based on observational studies that examine recurrent vascular events.[32] In addition to these studies,[111] the relation between hyperhomocysteinemia and carotid intima-media thickness has also been investigated in populations with confirmed or suspected vascular disease.

A beneficial effect of folic acid (2.5 mg), vitamin B_{12} (0.5 mg) and vitamin B_6 (25 mg) daily supplementation for one year on carotid intima-media thickness progression in patients with carotid intima-media thickness ≥1 mm has recently been demonstrated.[54] While homocysteine in the placebo group did not change during the course of the year, homocysteine decreased from 10.5±3.9 to 6.6±1.5 µmol/L in the active treatment group. Carotid intima-media thickness increased in the placebo group by 7.4±19.2% and decreased in the active treatment group by 4.2±12.8%. Differences in the rate of progression between the groups were detected at six months; increased carotid intima-media thickness responds quickly to high doses of oral B vitamin supplementation.

Seven observational studies have been conducted in individuals with suspected or confirmed cardiovascular complications as based on attendance to vascular disease screening programs or laboratories. The relation between homocysteine and carotid intima-media thickness was investigated in elderly Japanese men undergoing a cardiovascular examination.[174] When the group was stratified on the basis of hypertension prevalence, non-hypertensives had 5.8-fold increased odds for increased carotid intima-media thickness (third vs. first homocysteine tertile, 95% CI 1.24 to 27.1). Another study in elderly hospital patients demonstrated that carotid intima-media thickness increased per tertile increase in homocysteine.[171] In patients sent for vascular assessment with an carotid intima-media thickness ≥2 mm or <1.2 mm the odds of increased carotid intima-media thickness increased per unit increase in homocysteine (odds ratio [OR] 1.11, 95% CI 1.03 to 1.19).[173] Demuth and colleagues included attendees to a French cardiovascular risk factor screening program with a carotid intima-media thickness <1.0 mm.[176] Carotid intima-media thickness was positively associated with homocysteine, age, male gender and total cholesterol (R^2=0.291). A small study showed a positive correlation (r=0.5-0.7) in post-menopausal women with hypertension, although it is unclear if the investigators adjusted for other conventional risk factors for vascular disease.[177] The remaining two studies did not detect a positive relation between homocysteine and carotid intima-media thickness in neurological patients <55 years[170] or in patients referred for a transthoracic echocardiogram.[175]

Family members of individuals who develop vascular disease share genetic and environmental factors that increase vascular disease risk. A cross-sectional study has been conducted in family members of patients with vascular disease or increased carotid intima-media thickness.[172] In subjects ≥55 years only, carotid intima-media thickness was significantly greater in subjects with homocysteine ≥9.4 µmol/L compared with those with homocysteine <9.4 µmol/L.

In summary, often after examining effect modification (e.g. hypertension or older age), homocysteine was associated with carotid intima-media thickness. Subjects with suspected or confirmed vascular disease may have undergone dietary and lifestyle changes as a consequence of the vascular disease event, perhaps decreasing homocysteine levels. In contrast to the inconclusive observational studies, high doses of B vitamins led to a drastic and acute effect on carotid intima-media thickness. This trial needs to be confirmed and repeated in other types of vascular disease patients.

General population

Nine studies have been conducted in the general population with few inclusion criteria. The first study used baseline data from the Atherosclerosis Risk in Communities Study.[180] A homocysteine value in the highest quintile (>10.15 µmol/L) increased the likelihood 3.5-fold for having increased carotid intima-media thickness compared with the lowest quintile (<5.88 µmol/L) (paired OR 95% CI 1.57 to 6.33), however, after adjustment for confounders, the OR was no longer statistically significant. The adjusted OR for increased carotid intima-media thickness comparing the highest and lowest sex-specific homocysteine quartile was 2.60 (95% CI 1.51 to 4.45) in an Australian study.[179] In the Rotterdam Study, hyperhomocysteinemia (≥18.6 µmol/L) was associated with a 0.037 mm increase in carotid intima-media thickness (95% CI 0.0004 to 0.0740 mm) in subjects <75 years, however there was no association of homocysteine with carotid intima-media thickness in subjects ≥75 years.[181] In a Japanese farming community survey, homocysteine was an independent predictor of carotid intima-media thickness;[178] subjects in the third and fourth homocysteine quartiles showed a dose-dependent increase in carotid intima-media thickness compared with those below the median (<10.0 µmol/L). In a second Japanese study, the partial correlation coefficient for homocysteine and maximum carotid intima-media thickness ranged between 0.15-0.36 depending on C677T MTHFR genotype; in the same study, homocysteine was not correlated with mean carotid intima-media thickness.[185] Finally, homocysteine was not associated with either mean or maximum carotid intima-media thickness in British, French or Dutch populations.[85,182-184] In conclusion, the association between homocysteine and carotid intima-media thickness in the general population is often weak or absent.

Homocysteine is an independent risk factor in two studies conducted in healthy populations. In Italian postmenopausal women who met stringent inclusion criteria, a 10 µmol/L increase in homocysteine was not associated with an increased likelihood of having increased carotid intima-media thickness (>1 mm); however, when carotid intima-media thickness was analyzed as a continuous variable, 29% of the variation in carotid intima-media thickness was attributed to homocysteine.[186] Likewise, in a German study of 75 healthy men and women, after adjustment for age, body mass index and LDL cholesterol, the addition of homocysteine in the regression model explained approximately 18% of the variation in adjusted carotid intima-media thickness.[187]

5,10-Methylenetetrahydrofolate reductase 677C→T polymorphism

The most common genetic determinant of hyperhomocysteinemia in the general population is a C to T substitution at nucleotide 677 in the gene encoding MTHFR. Carriers of the MTHFR 677T allele have a decreased specific activity to reduce 5,10-methylenetetrahydrofolate to 5-methyltetrahydrofolate[202] probably due to the destabilization of the coenzyme, flavin adenine dinucleotide.[203] The polymorphism modulates homocysteine response to folate.[204]

Data from a pooled analysis of almost 30,000 cases of coronary heart disease and controls have shown that having the MTHFR 677TT genotype confer a 16% increase in risk (95% CI 1.06 to 1.27).[78] Although this meta-analysis is viewed as a mainstay for the possible pathogenic role of homocysteine in vascular disease, reduced activity of MTHFR does not lead solely to hyperhomocysteinemia when folate status is low. MTHFR is involved in other enzymatic pathways such as the reduction of quinonoid dihydropterins,[205] specifically the formation of tetrahydrobiopterin may be important for endothelial nitric oxide synthase activity.[206] Furthermore, the distribution of folate derivatives in TT carriers is shifted: an increase in formylated methyl folates important for purine synthesis and a decrease in 5-methyltetrahydrofolate[207] important for *S*-adenosylmethionine biosynthesis and possibly tetrahydrobiopterin binding to endothelial nitric oxide synthase.[208] Thus, polymorphic MTHFR has several effects that could explain the increased risk of vascular disease conferred to MTHFR 677TT carriers.

Seven out of fourteen studies reported a positive association of MTHFR 677TT genotype or 677T allele frequency with extent of arterial thickening.[151,186,209-212] Two of these studies simultaneously investigated the association of homocysteine and MTHFR polymorphism with carotid intima-media thickness, which has led to inconsistent results.[151,186] The unexpected finding in which MTHFR and not homocysteine was associated with carotid intima-media thickness may be explained by the standard B vitamin therapy given to this end-stage renal disease patient population.[151] The remaining studies failed to show an association of MTHFR 677TT genotype with carotid intima-media thickness.[162,163,169,176,179,185,213] Three studies demonstrated an relation between homocysteine and carotid intima-media thickness but not between MTHFR and carotid intima-media thickness.[176,179,185]

It is likely that the MTHFR polymorphism is associated with carotid intima-media thickness. An adequate sample size is needed to explore this association properly in future research. Furthermore, no studies reported on the attenuation of the association of the MTHFR C677T genotype with carotid intima-media thickness when homocysteine is entered into the statistical model or to explore the effect of MTHFR in low folate groups.

Folate status

Beneficial effects of folate on vascular disease have conventionally been attributed to its homocysteine-lowering ability. However, folate has antioxidant properties that enhance the endothelial atheroprotective phenotype by scavenging superoxide radicals and potentiating tetrahydrobiopterin in its role as a coenzyme for endothelial nitric oxide synthase.[208] Folate deficiency triggers NF-κB activation,[214] and in apoE deficient mice, hyperhomocysteinemic-induced NF-κB activity is decreased when extra B vitamins are supplemented.[215] Cohort and case-cohort studies suggest that low folate intake[34-37] and low levels of serum or erythrocyte folate,[36-45] independent of homocysteine,[37-39] are associated with vascular disease morbidity and mortality; however, many of the risk estimates did not reach statistical significance. In contrast, in an elderly cohort followed for approximately six years, no association was demonstrated with folate status and mortality.[216]

All studies but one[183] found no association of folate status with carotid intima-media thickness,[163,165,173,186,187] even when analysis was confined to the lowest folate values.[179] Normal folate levels in the populations studied may explain the lack of association with carotid intima-media thickness; perhaps a threshold of folate deficiency must be attained before such an association can be found.

Discussion

Homocysteine was not related to carotid intima-media thickness in homocystinuric, uremic, cholesterolemic or non-insulin dependent diabetes mellitus patients nor in subjects with insulin insensitivity. It is possible that risk factors associated with these disorders mask a weaker association of homocysteine with carotid intima-media thickness, as probably is the case in familial hypercholesterolemia patients (Figure 2.3). In the case of homocystinuria, the nature of atherogenesis may differ from the general population due to broader amino acid disturbances. In uremic populations hyperhomocysteinemia is mainly a secondary phenomenon of renal dysfunction and may not directly relate to atherogenesis. In vascular disease patients and in the general population homocysteine is weakly related to carotid intima-media thickness, often only after stratifying the population based on e.g. hypertension, age and sex or in populations screened on stringent health criteria. Evidence from trials in renal transplant recipients and vascular disease patients showing that B vitamins supplementation leads to carotid intima-media thickness regression certainly offer a beacon of hope for these patient groups.

Combining this evidence, homocysteine may be involved in the early stages (i.e. atherosclerosis) and advanced stages of vascular disease (i.e. lesion instability, neointimal hyperplasia, thrombosis). It is unlikely that homocysteine is merely a reflection of atherosclerotic damage, as one would expect higher homocysteine in individuals with greatly increased carotid intima-media thickness as in familial hypercholesterolemia. We cannot disregard the possibility that hyperhomocysteinemia is an epiphenomenon of renal dysfunction or is an 'innocent' covariate of a disturbed methylation process. In contrast to the often inconclusive evidence from the observational studies, acute and rather strong beneficial effects on carotid intima-media thickness from high doses of folic acid, vitamin B_6 and vitamin B_{12} have been demonstrated in two high-risk populations. However, strictly speaking, the culprit—hyperhomocysteinemia or low levels of B vitamins—leading to increased carotid intima-media thickness can not be teased out from these B vitamin trials; trials using methylation enhancers which do not affect homocysteine levels (i.e. betaine, serine, *S*-adenosylmethionine) are needed to answer this question. Although most studies have not found an association of folate with carotid intima-media thickness, it is possible that low folate concentrations are weakly associated with carotid intima-media thickness. Studies including subjects with suboptimal folate levels need to be conducted. Data from studies suffering from power problems show that the MTHFR 677TT genotype is generally positively associated with carotid intima-media thickness. Larger studies and pooled analyses are needed to determine if MTHFR C677T polymorphism is indeed associated with carotid intima-

Table 2.3 Overview of on-going homocysteine-lowering trials using carotid intima-media thickness as an endpoint.[a]

	FACIT[48]	DIVINe[b]
Homocysteine-lowering regime	0.8 mg folic acid	2.5 mg folic acid, 25 mg B_6, 1 mg B_{12}
Duration of trial	3 y	2 y
Number of participants	819	122
Main eligibility criteria	50-70 y, homocysteine ≥13 μmol/L	NIDDM/IDDM, diabetic nephropathy
Intima-media thickness outcome	Mean and max CCA	Mean CCA
Intima-media thickness protocol	R & L distal CCA, FW & NW	R & L distal CCA, FW
Other endpoints of atherosclerosis	Carotid arterial stiffness Carotid plaque area[c]	Carotid plaque progression

[a] Abbreviations. FACIT Folic Acid and Carotid Intima-media Thickness trial; DIVINe the Diabetic Intervention with Vitamins to Improve Nephropathy trial; NIDDM non-insulin dependent diabetes mellitus; IDDM insulin dependent diabetes mellitus; CCA common carotid artery; R right; L left; FW far wall; NW near wall.
[b] A House. Personal communication.
[c] Measurement added after original publication.

media thickness. Nonetheless, these preliminary findings support a role of folate or homocysteine in atherosclerosis and vascular disease.

Various carotid intima-media thickness methodologies were employed which impedes a meta-analysis based on the results of these studies. This has been a source of critique as to the usefulness of carotid intima-media thickness as a surrogate measure of vascular disease (Table 2.2).[217] Consensus should be reached to create a standardized carotid intima-media thickness protocol to facilitate the use, comparison and interpretation of carotid intima-media thickness as a surrogate marker. Consensus is required if one is interested in the segment-specific susceptibility to hyperhomocysteinemia or in local carotid atherosclerosis *per se*. Since carotid intima-media thickness in all segments predict future disease equally well,[218] carotid intima-media thickness, used as a marker for risk, is not greatly affected by between study differences in methods.

Results from homocysteine-lowering trials using carotid intima-media thickness as an outcome offer necessary but not conclusive evidence for the causality of homocysteine in atherosclerosis. Two trials, one in hyperhomocysteinemic elderly and the other in patients with diabetic nephropathy, are underway (Table 2.3). However, carotid intima-media thickness may not fully capture arterial changes due to homocysteine-lowering. Although the total arterial wall is involved in atherosclerosis, the intima has been the primary arterial wall of interest. Carotid intima-media thickness is dominated by the medial thickness, the percentage of which decreases as atherosclerosis progresses.[217]

Arterial morphology associated with hyperhomocysteinemia in animal studies give conflicting results on the medial wall[219-221] whereas in humans this area has remained relatively unexplored.[129,221] The only morphological distinction between peripheral arterial disease patients with and without hyperhomocysteinemia was a decreased medial smooth muscle cell / extracellular matrix ratio, which may lead to a decrease in arterial compliance.[221] Unfortunately, comparison of the intimal wall between the two groups of cardiovascular disease patients was not possible. Whether these findings in often-occluded biopsies of the muscular femoral artery may be extrapolated to other arterial beds including the elastic carotid artery remains to be determined. In conclusion, trials using markers of atherosclerosis should consider a combination of structural and functional parameters until the mechanisms of pathogenesis of hyperhomocysteinemia are solved.

The mechanisms through which hyperhomocysteinemia promote vascular disease remain an active area of research. Hyperhomocysteinemia leads to increased oxidative stress via the generation of reactive oxygen species which weaken intracellular anti-oxidation defense systems[222] or elicit intracellular redox controlled inflammation responses.[223] From cell and animal studies a variety of putative responses which enhance atherosclerosis or evoke its complications are thought to stem from the homocysteine-mediated oxidative stress hypothesis: inhibition of nitric oxide synthesis and/or bioavailability;[224,225] proliferation of smooth muscle cell;[226] modification of LDL cholesterol;[227] intimal and neointimal hyperplasia;[219,227,228] increased protease[219,228] activity;[215,229] activation of NF-κB and proinflammatory markers;[215] and thrombosis.[215,230] Other pathogenic mechanisms of homocysteine independent of the 'oxidative stress' theory, such as generation of homocysteine thiolactone and associated protein homocysteinylation[231] and generation of asymmetric dimethylarginine, an endogenous inhibitor of nitric oxide synthase,[232] are currently under investigation. Benefits of homocysteine reduction for primary prevention in hyperhomocysteinemic animal models include a decreased inflammation and prothrombotic response and increased plaque stability,[215] but effects on vessel lesion progression[215,233] and thickness of the intimal and medial arterial wall[220,233] are inconsistent. Findings relevant for secondary prevention studies suggest that folic acid treatment decreases neointimal formation in a rat balloon injury model[219] and luminal stenosis in a rat endarterectomy model.[234]

Well-designed trials are needed to disentangle the possible causal role of hyperhomocysteinemia in relation to vascular disease. B vitamin therapy slows down atherogenesis in vascular disease patients as measured by progression of carotid plaque area,[62,63] however, the effects of B vitamin on rate of coronary restenosis have been contradictory[52,53] and in uremic patients B vitamin therapy did not affect arterial stiffness.[91] In the general population, two-year allocation to B vitamin therapy compared with placebo therapy showed a protective effect for normal exercise electrocardiography test but failed to demonstrate a beneficial effect on carotid or femoral stenosis or ankle-brachial index.[56] Large-scale randomized placebo-controlled clinical trials, which test the effects B vitamins on vascular disease hard endpoints are underway.[235] The first reports are disheartening and some are still to be published. In general, no discernible effects of B vitamins on the risk of reoccurring cardiovascular events have been found.[59,65] Many of these intervention studies may lack power to confirm or refute the homocysteine hypothesis; however a future meta-analysis of the evidence from these studies and surrogate marker studies relevant for the general population is especially pertinent in light of emerging health claims on the protective role of B vitamins in vascular disease.[51]

Chapter 3

Low concentrations of folate, not hyperhomocysteinemia, are associated with increased carotid intima-media thickness

Jane Durga, Michiel L. Bots, Evert G. Schouten, Frans J. Kok, Petra Verhoef

Division of Human Nutrition, Wageningen University, Wageningen, The Netherlands
Wageningen Centre for Food Sciences, Wageningen, The Netherlands
Julius Center for Health Sciences and Primary Care, University Medical Center Utrecht, Utrecht, The Netherlands

Submitted

Abstract

Aim We examined whether total homocysteine, B vitamins and the 5,10-methylenetetrahydrofolate reductase (MTHFR) 677C→T polymorphism are related to common carotid intima-media thickness, a marker of atherosclerosis, and carotid distension, a marker of arterial stiffness.

Methods We used cross-sectional data from 819 individuals aged 50 to 70 years. B-mode ultrasound of the distal common carotid arteries was performed to determine maximum carotid intima-media thickness, mean carotid intima-media thickness and distension.

Results Carotid intima-media thickness and distension did not differ across homocysteine, serum folate, vitamin B_6 and vitamin B_{12} quartiles or between MTHFR C677T genotype. Erythrocyte folate was independently associated with maximum carotid intima-media thickness (mean difference first vs. third quartile, 0.03 mm, 95% CI 0.004 to 0.06 mm; first vs. fourth quartile, 0.03 mm, 95% CI -0.002 to 0.06 mm). Further adjustment for homocysteine did not affect this association. Folate deficient subjects had greater maximum carotid intima-media thickness than those with high-normal folate concentrations (serum folate: mean difference 0.05 mm, 95% CI 0.01 to 0.08 mm; erythrocyte folate: mean difference 0.04 mm, 95% CI -0.03 to 0.11 mm).

Conclusion Low folate concentrations, independent of hyperhomocysteinemia, may promote atherogenesis. Our findings confirm the null association of homocysteine with carotid intima-media thickness observed in other population-based studies, suggesting that hyperhomocysteinemia does not perpetuate atherosclerosis or arterial stiffness.

Introduction

An elevated level of plasma total homocysteine, or hyperhomocysteinemia, is an independent risk factor for vascular disease.[236] Likewise, determinants of hyperhomocysteinemia, such as low concentrations of B vitamin coenzymes involved in homocysteine metabolism and a C→T mutation at the 677 base pair of the methylenetetrahydrofolate reductase (MTHFR) gene, are also associated with increased risk of vascular disease.[36,78,237] It is unclear whether hyperhomocysteinemia or low concentrations of B vitamins are atherogenic *per se* or conduce factors that trigger vascular disease to occur in the presence of atherosclerosis (e.g. imbalance in hemostasis).

A recent review has summarized more than fifty studies that have examined the association of homocysteine with carotid intima-media thickness,[238] a marker of atherosclerosis and a valid surrogate marker of vascular disease.[239] Few studies conducted in the general population have demonstrated weak positive associations between homocysteine and carotid intima-media thickness, and often only in sub-samples such as normotensives[174] or men.[161] In contrast, folate status or intake, vitamins B_{12} and B_6 status and the C677T MTHFR polymorphism have not been associated with carotid intima-media thickness in the general population.[238] These findings may in part be due to small sample sizes and the adequate B vitamin status in the study populations.

Arterial stiffness has been less utilized in epidemiological research. Arterial stiffness has been associated with age-related arterial changes, atherosclerosis and vascular disease.[240] Studies have reported null associations of homocysteine with arterial stiffness in the general population.[85,87,143,241] A small study conducted in women demonstrated that MTHFR 677TT homozygotes had higher end diastolic velocity of the common carotid artery (n=120),[186] however, a larger study has shown no relation between MTHFR 677T allele frequency and aortic pulse wave velocity (n=1160).[85] No studies to our knowledge have reported on the association of B vitamins with arterial stiffness in the general population.

In this paper we test the hypothesis that elevated homocysteine, MTHFR 677TT genotype, and low concentrations of B vitamins constitute risk factors for atherosclerosis, as measured by common carotid intima-media thickness and carotid distension, in older subjects with increased concentrations of homocysteine.

Methods

Subjects

Data are from 819 men and post-menopausal women aged 50 to 70 years who were participating in the Folic Acid and Carotid Intima-media Thickness (FACIT) study, a trial investigating whether folic acid supplementation can halt the progression of atherosclerosis. Major exclusion criteria were homocysteine <13 µmol/L, vitamin B_{12} <200 pmol/L, no renal or thyroid diseases and no current use of B vitamin supplements or medications that influence folate metabolism or carotid intima-media thickness progression (e.g. lipid-lowering and hormone replacement therapies). The Medical Ethics Committee of Wageningen University approved the study and subjects gave written informed consent.

Blood measurements

Fasting venous blood was collected, directly processed and stored at -80°C until determination. Erythrocyte and serum folate and serum vitamin B_{12} were measured using a chemiluminescent immunoassay (Immulite® 2000, Diagnostic Products Corporation). Erythrocyte folate was determined in duplicate. Plasma homocysteine was determined with HPLC and fluorimetric detection.[242] Serum creatinine and lipids were determined using Hitachi® 747 (Roche). We defined hypercholesterolemia as total cholesterol >6.5 mmol/L, high-density lipoprotein cholesterol <0.9 mmol/L or use of lipid-lowering medication. Vitamin B_6 was measured by HPLC. C-reactive protein was determined with ELISA using polyclonal antibodies (Dako). The C677T MTHFR genotype was determined by PCR of DNA and restriction enzyme digestion with *Hin*Fl. Intra and inter assay variation coefficients for laboratory analyses were <15%.

Carotid ultrasound

High-resolution B-mode carotid ultrasonography was performed with a 7.5 MHz linear-array transducer (ATL UltraMark IX). In a dark quiet room the subject was in supine position with his head tilted 45° in the direction opposite of the carotid being measured. Longitudinal images of the distal common carotid arteries were obtained at four predefined angles of 30° steps (90° to 180° on the right side and 270° to 180° on the left side). Images were frozen on the top of the R-wave of the electrocardiography and recorded on VHS tape. The mean and mean of the maximum distance of the near and far wall of the distal 10 mm of the right and left common carotid arteries was determined using an automated edge detection program. Lumen diameter was estimated as the mean distance between the leading edge of the intima-lumen interface and the lumen-intima interface. At an angle deemed by the sonographer to give the best visualization of the arterial walls, an M-line was placed at the measurement site. In M-mode, the sonographer recorded carotid artery pulsation for approximately three seconds. The relative distension of the carotid artery was calculated as the absolute change in lumen diameter relative to its end-diastolic diameter was calculated. The average of three measurements per side was calculated.

Ultrasound examination was performed in duplicate within three weeks; the average was used for analyses. The same sonographer performed both examinations in 91% of the subjects. A single reader interpreted all images. The mean difference (± standard deviation [SD]) between the sonographers was 0.09 mm (±0.10 mm) for maximum carotid intima-media thickness, 0.05 mm (±0.04 mm) for mean carotid intima-media thickness and 0.02 mm (±0.03 mm) for distension. The intraclass correlation coefficient for maximum carotid intima-media thickness was 0.90 for sonographer 1 and 0.88 for sonographer 2, for mean carotid intima-media thickness was 0.96 for both sonographers and for distension was 0.77 for sonographer 1 and 0.88 for sonographer 2. Both sonographers and the reader were blinded to participants' homocysteine values.

Other measurements

A self-reported medical history, smoking and physical activity habits[243] were attained by questionnaire and reviewed by a trained research assistant. A participant was considered to have prevalent vascular disease if he had been diagnosed with angina pectoris, myocardial infarction, arrhythmia, stroke, or peripheral arterial disease or if he had undergone certain palliative procedures (balloon angioplasty, coronary bypass surgery or aortic aneurysm surgery). Height and weight were measured and body mass index (BMI) (kg/m^2) was calculated. Blood pressure was measured using an automated meter (Dinamap® Compact Pro 100, General Electric) in supine position, while the participant underwent the ultrasound examination. The average of eight measurements was taken. We defined hypertension as systolic blood pressure ≥160 mmHg, diastolic blood pressure ≥95 mmHg or use of antihypertensive medication. Mean arterial pressure was calculated by the following formula: diastolic blood pressure + 1/3 · (systolic blood pressure – diastolic blood pressure). A food frequency questionnaire estimated folate intake and alcohol intake in the past three months. Food items and portion sizes used by men and women aged 50 to 70 years were derived from the Dutch Nutrition Survey.[244] Two typists, blinded to study information, separately entered all data.

Statistical analysis

Statistical analyses were performed using SPSS 11.0 for Windows. Depending on the distribution of the variable, results are expressed as mean ± SD or median (interquartile range). We performed multivariate regression analyses adjusted for sex and age to determine the linear relationship between independent variables and carotid intima-media thickness. Univariate general linear model was used to calculate maximum and mean carotid intima-media thickness and distension per quartile of homocysteine and B vitamins, per B vitamin deficiency status and per MTHFR C677T genotype. Initially, crude associations were examined. Age and sex, and then risk factors for vascular disease (lipids, blood pressure, creatinine, use of antihypertensive or lipid-lowering therapy, current smoking status, smoking pack-years, body mass index and prevalence of diabetes mellitus) were subsequently added to the regression models. Because of the high correlation between diastolic blood pressure, systolic blood pressure and mean arterial pressure and between low-density lipoprotein (LDL) cholesterol and total cholesterol we entered systolic blood pressure and LDL cholesterol in models for carotid intima-media thickness and mean arterial pressure and LDL cholesterol in models for distension (r_S>0.90). To investigate if elevated concentrations of homocysteine or C-reactive protein may mediate the association between low B vitamins and carotid intima-media thickness and distension, we subsequently entered homocysteine and C-reactive protein in the model. We used the Kruskal-Wallis test, followed by the Mann Whitney test to determine whether MTHFR 677T allele frequency was associated with high concentrations of homocysteine and low concentrations of folate. Only age and sex adjusted analyses were conducted when studying the association between MTHFR C677T genotype and carotid intima-media thickness. Because the MTHFR 677T allele is associated with hyperhomocysteinemia when folate status is low, we stratified the population based on folate status. Statistical significance was defined as $p<0.05$ (two-tailed).

Results

Characteristics of the population are shown in Table 3.1. The median homocysteine concentration in this population was 12.9 µmol/L (interquartile range 11.5 to 14.7 µmol/L). The median homocysteine and vitamin B_{12} of the population at baseline were lower than at screening. The low correlation between screening and study values of homocysteine and vitamin B_{12} indicates high intra-individual variability (homocysteine r_S=0.49 [95% CI 0.41 to 0.54], vitamin B_{12} r_S=0.77 [95% CI 0.74 to 0.80]). Therefore, we

Table 3.1 Characteristics of study population (*n*=819).

		Mean (standard deviation) Median (interquartile range)
Demographics		
	Age, years	60 ± 6
	% Male	72
Markers of vascular disease		
	Mean carotid intima-media thickness, mm	0.83 ± 0.13
	Maximum carotid intima-media thickness, mm	1.02 ± 0.17
	Carotid distension, mm	0.63 ± 0.17
	Lumen diameter, mm	6.09 (5.66 to 6.63)
	Lumen diameter for distension, mm	6.23 (5.75 to 6.81)
	Mean arterial pressure, mmHg	100 ± 11
	% Vascular disease	12
Clinical		
	Homocysteine, study commencement, µmol/L	12.9 (11.5 to 14.7)
	Mean homocysteine, screening & study commencement, µmol/L	13.8 (12.8 to 15.4)
	% 5,10-methylenetetrahydrofolate reductase 677 CC / CT / TT	38 / 47 / 15
	Serum folate, nmol/L	12 (10 to 15)
	Erythrocyte folate, nmol/L	659 (515 to 818)
	Vitamin B_{12}, pmol/L	289 (242 to 264)
	Vitamin B_6, nmol/L	32 (24 to 42)
	Creatinine, µmol/L	93 ± 12
	Total cholesterol, mmol/L	5.8 ± 1.1
	High-density lipoprotein cholesterol, mmol/L	1.2 ± 0.4
	Low-density lipoprotein cholesterol, mmol/L	4.0 ± 1.0
	Triglycerides, mmol/L	1.2 (0.8 to 1.6)
	% Hypercholesterolemia	36
	Systolic blood pressure, mmHg	133 ± 16
	Diastolic blood pressure, mmHg	77 ± 8
	% Hypertension	22
	C-reactive protein, mg/L	1.11 (0.59 to 2.31)
	Body mass index, kg/m^2	27 ± 4
	% Diabetes mellitus	3
Lifestyle		
	% Current smokers	20
	Folate intake, µg/d	194 (159 to 240)
	Alcohol intake, g/d	13 (4 to 24)

used the mean of screening and study values for further analyses. The prevalence of erythrocyte folate, serum folate or vitamin B_6 deficiency was 2.4%, 8.9% and 13.2%, respectively (cut-off: erythrocyte folate ≤305 nmol/L, serum folate ≤7 nmol/L, vitaminB_6 ≤20 nmol/L).[245] The MTHFR 677T allelic distribution did not significantly

Table 3.2 Age and sex adjusted partial correlation coefficients of maximum carotid intima-media thickness and carotid distension (*n*=819).

Variables[a]	Partial correlation coefficient: Maximum intima-media thickness	Distension
Age	0.40*	-0.08*
Sex	0.22*	0.02
Lumen diameter	0.40*	0.01
Mean arterial pressure	0.19*	-0.03
Homocysteine	0.04	-0.01
5,10-methylenetetrahydrofolate reductase 677C→T	0.02	0.01
Serum folate	-0.02	0.03
Erythrocyte folate	-0.05	0.01
Vitamin B_{12}	0.01	0.01
Vitamin B_6	-0.08*	0.01
Folate intake	0.08*	0.02
Alcohol intake	-0.08*	0.04
Creatinine	0.07*	-0.08*
Total cholesterol	0.04	-0.04
High-density lipoprotein cholesterol	-0.13*	0.01
Low-density lipoprotein cholesterol	0.06	-0.04
Triglycerides	0.09*	-0.02
Hypercholesterolemia	0.11*	0.02
Systolic blood pressure	0.28*	0.10*
Diastolic blood pressure	0.09*	-0.13*
Hypertension	0.16*	-0.02
C-reactive protein	0.05	0.05
Body mass index	0.15*	-0.06
Current smoking	0.03	0.02
Smoking pack-years	0.15*	0.04
Vascular disease	0.14*	0.02
Diabetes mellitus	0.16*	0.01

* $p<0.05$.
[a] Variables coded 0. Women, MTHFR 677CC genotype, no hypertension nor hypercholesterolemia, never smoker, no vascular disease or diabetes mellitus.

differ from the calculated expected distribution, assuming a Hardy-Weinberg equilibrium. The percentage of MTHFR 677TT genotype (15%) was higher than in the general Dutch population (10%),[39] a likely consequence of our homocysteine inclusion criteria.

Although maximum and mean carotid intima-media thickness were highly correlated (r_p=0.91, $p<0.001$) and shared similar risk factors, the association between the explanatory variables and carotid intima-media thickness was generally stronger for maximum carotid intima-media thickness than mean carotid intima-media thickness. Distension was correlated with maximum and mean carotid intima-media thickness (r_S=0.11, p=0.002, r_S=0.16, p<0.001 respectively) but with few other variables (Table 3.2). Age, sex and body mass index were independent determinants of distension (data not shown). However, neither homocysteine nor the B vitamins were related to distension (Table 3.3).

Maximum carotid intima-media thickness in subjects in the upper quartile of the homocysteine distribution was average 0.04 mm greater than those in the lowest homocysteine quartile (95% CI 0.01 to 0.08 mm). After adjusting for age and sex or additional confounders, maximum carotid intima-media thickness did not differ substantially between the homocysteine quartiles (Table 3.3).

When the population was divided into quartiles of B vitamin status, belonging to the lowest quartile of serum folate (≤9 nmol/L) was not paired with a greater mean or maximum carotid intima-media thickness in either crude or adjusted analyses (Table 3.3). Subjects in the lowest erythrocyte folate quartile (≤514 nmol/L) had slightly greater maximum carotid intima-media thickness than the rest of the population. Differences in carotid intima-media thickness between the erythrocyte folate quartiles increased after adjustment for age and sex. After adjustment for confounders, differences weakened but remained statistically significant (first vs. third quartile, 0.03 mm, 95% CI 0.004 to 0.06 mm; first vs. fourth quartile, 0.03 mm, 95% CI -0.002 to 0.06 mm). Further adjustment for homocysteine or C-reactive protein concentrations did not affect this association. Similarly, in crude and age and sex adjusted analyses, subjects in the lowest quartile of vitamin B_6 had a greater carotid intima-media thickness than subjects in the highest quartile. This association disappeared when confounders were entered into the regression model. Finally, vitamin B_{12} concentrations were not associated with carotid intima-media thickness, although subjects in the highest tertile of the vitamin B_{12} distribution tended to have increased carotid intima-media thickness in all analyses.

To examine whether B vitamins needed to reach a critical low before an association between the B vitamins and carotid intima-media thickness can be detected, we stratified the population based on B vitamin deficiency. Subjects deficient in either serum or erythrocyte folate had on average a greater maximum carotid intima-media thickness than those with high-normal folate concentrations (mean difference adjusted for age and sex: serum folate deficient vs. low-normal 0.05 mm, 95% CI 0.01 to 0.09 mm, deficient

Table 3.3 Mean values of maximum carotid intima-media thickness (CIMT) and carotid distension in mm per homocysteine and B vitamin quartile and per folate status, adjusted for age and sex (*n*=819).

	Maximum intima-media thickness and distension (95% confidence interval)				P_{trend}
Quartiles[a]	1	2	3	4	
Homocysteine					
Maximum CIMT	1.01 (0.99 to 1.03)	1.03 (1.01 to 1.05)	1.02 (1.00 to 1.04)	1.03 (1.00 to 1.05)	0.254
Distension	0.62 (0.60 to 0.64)	0.64 (0.61 to 0.66)	0.65 (0.62 to 0.67)	0.63 (0.61 to 0.65)	0.808
Serum folate					
Maximum CIMT	1.03 (1.01 to 1.05)	1.01 (0.99 to 1.03)	1.01 (0.99 to 1.03)	1.03 (1.01 to 1.05)	0.501
Distension	0.63 (0.61 to 0.65)	0.63 (0.61 to 0.65)	0.64 (0.62 to 0.66)	0.64 (0.61 to 0.66)	0.420
Erythrocyte folate					
Maximum CIMT	1.05 (1.03 to 1.07)	1.02 (0.99 to 1.04)	1.01 (0.98 to 1.03)	1.01 (0.99 to 1.03)	0.184
Distension	0.63 (0.61 to 0.65)	0.64 (0.62 to 0.66)	0.64 (0.62 to 0.66)	0.62 (0.60 to 0.65)	0.845
Vitamin B_{12}					
Maximum CIMT	1.01 (0.99 to 1.03)	1.01 (0.99 to 1.03)	1.03 (1.01 to 1.05)	1.03 (1.01 to 1.06)	0.344
Distension	0.62 (0.60 to 0.64)	0.64 (0.61 to 0.66)	0.64 (0.61 to 0.66)	0.64 (0.62 to 0.66)	0.840
Vitamin B_6					
Maximum CIMT	1.04 (1.02 to 1.06)	1.01 (0.99 to 1.03)	1.03 (1.01 to 1.04)	1.00 (0.98 to 1.03)	0.028
Distension	0.63 (0.60 to 0.65)	0.64 (0.62 to 0.66)	0.63 (0.61 to 0.65)	0.64 (0.62 to 0.66)	0.773

Vitamin status[b]	Deficient		Low-normal		High-normal	
Serum folate						
Maximum CIMT	1.04	(1.01 to 1.08)	1.02	(1.00 to 1.03)	1.02	(1.01 to 1.03)
Distension	0.62	(0.58 to 0.66)	0.63	(0.61 to 0.65)	0.64	(0.62 to 0.66)
Erythrocyte folate						
Maximum CIMT	1.06	(0.99 to 1.12)	1.05	(1.02 to 1.07)	1.01	(1.00 to 1.03)
Distension	0.59	(0.52 to 0.67)	0.64	(0.61 to 0.66)	0.63	(0.62 to 0.65)
Vitamin B_6 status						
Maximum CIMT	1.04	(1.01 to 1.07)	1.02	(1.00 to 1.04)	1.02	(1.00 to 1.03)
Distension	0.63	(0.60 to 0.66)	0.63	(0.61 to 0.66)	0.63	(0.62 to 0.65)

[a] Quartile cut-off (upper limit). Homocysteine ≤11.5 μmol/L, 12.9 μmol/L, 14.6 μmol/L; Serum folate ≤9 nmol/L, 11 nmol/L, 14 nmol/L; Erythrocyte folate ≤514 nmol/L, 659 nmol/L, 817 nmol/L; Vitamin B_{12} ≤242 pmol/L, 288 pmol/L, 364 pmol/L; Vitamin B_6 ≤24 nmol/L, 31 nmol/L, 41 nmol/L.

[b] Serum folate status: Deficient ≤7 nmol/L, *n*=73; Low-normal 8-11 nmol/L, *n*=319; High-normal ≥12 nmol/L, *n*=427. Erythrocyte folate status: Deficient ≤305 nmol/L, *n*=20; Low-normal 306-500 nmol/L, *n*=169; High-normal ≥501 nmol/L, *n*=630. Vitamin B_6 status: Deficient ≤20 nmol/L, *n*=108; Low-normal 21-30 nmol/L, *n*=255; High-normal ≥31 nmol/L, *n*=456.

vs. high-normal 0.05 mm 95% CI 0.01 to 0.08 mm; erythrocyte folate deficient vs. high-normal 0.04 mm, 95% CI -0.03 to 0.11 mm, low-normal vs. high-normal 0.03 mm, 95% CI 0.01 to 0.06 mm) (Table 3.3). Differences weakened and were no longer statistically significant after adjustment for confounders. Subjects with vitamin B_6 deficiency did not have an increased carotid intima-media thickness.

Subjects with the MTHFR 677TT genotype had on average greater homocysteine and lower folate concentrations than subjects with the MTHFR 677CC genotype, even though folate intake was similar between genotypes (data not shown). The MTHFR 677T allele was not associated with increased carotid intima-media thickness or decreased distension (Table 3.4).

Discussion

In our study folate deficiency was associated with increased carotid intima-media thickness, a marker of atherosclerosis and vascular disease. This is the first report showing an inverse association between folate and carotid intima-media thickness, probably because we included subjects in our study with suboptimal folate status. Furthermore, the association between folate and carotid intima-media thickness was independent of homocysteine. Homocysteine, on the other hand, was associated with carotid intima-media thickness in crude analyses but not after adjustment for risk factors of vascular disease. Our study had enough power (β=0.20) to detect a correlation of r=0.10 between homocysteine and carotid intima-media thickness, three-fold lower in magnitude than correlations published from other studies conducted in the general population with similar homocysteine median and homocysteine variance as our own study.[178,185] Vitamin B_6 and vitamin B_{12} were not independently associated with carotid intima-media thickness or distension, in agreement with other reports.[179,186,238]

The association between homocysteine and maximum and mean carotid intima-media thickness in the general population is absent in The Netherlands and weak worldwide.[238] Some investigators found an association after stratifying their population based on risk factor prevalence. In a Finnish population-based study a positive association between homocysteine and carotid intima-media thickness (0.01 mm difference in carotid intima-media thickness between homocysteine <11.5 μmol/L and ≥11.5 μmol/L) in men but not in women was found.[161] When we stratified the population based on sex, homocysteine was not associated with carotid intima-media thickness in men whereas women in the highest homocysteine quartile had on average 0.05 mm greater carotid

Table 3.4 Mean values of maximum carotid intima-media thickness (CIMT) and carotid distension in mm per MTHFR 677C→T genotype stratified by folate status, adjusted for age and sex.

	Mean (95% confidence interval)						P_{trend}
MTHFR 677C→T genotype	CC		CT		TT		
Serum folate[a]							
<50 percentile							
Maximum CIMT	1.00	(0.98 to 1.03)	1.03	(1.00 to 1.05)	1.03	(1.00 to 1.07)	0.378
Distension	0.62	(0.59 to 0.64)	0.64	(0.62 to 0.66)	0.64	(0.60 to 0.67)	0.373
>50 percentile							
Maximum CIMT	1.03	(1.01 to 1.06)	1.01	(0.99 to 1.04)	1.03	(0.98 to 1.07)	0.497
Distension	0.64	(0.61 to 0.67)	0.64	(0.62 to 0.67)	0.62	(0.57 to 0.67)	0.806
Erythrocyte folate[b]							
<50 percentile							
Maximum CIMT	1.03	(1.00 to 1.05)	1.03	(1.01 to 1.05)	1.05	(1.01 to 1.09)	0.634
Distension	0.62	(0.59 to 0.65)	0.65	(0.63 to 0.67)	0.63	(0.59 to 0.67)	0.314
>50 percentile							
Maximum CIMT	1.02	(0.99 to 1.04)	1.01	(0.98 to 1.03)	1.02	(0.98 to 1.06)	0.828
Distension	0.64	(0.61 to 0.66)	0.63	(0.60 to 0.66)	0.63	(0.59 to 0.67)	0.947

[a] Serum folate. <50 percentile (≤11.7 nmol/L) CC *n*=144, CT *n*=192, TT *n*=76; >50 percentile CC *n*=168, CT *n*=186, TT *n*=49.

[b] Erythrocyte folate. <50 percentile (≤659 nmol/L) CC *n*=133, CT *n*=215, TT *n*=59; >50 percentile CC *n*=179, CT *n*=163, TT *n*=66.

intima-media thickness (95% CI 0.001 to 0.11 mm, P_{trend}=0.032) compared with women in the lowest quartile (data not shown). In Japan, Okamura and colleagues detected a significant relationship between homocysteine and increased carotid intima-media thickness in normotensives (odds ratio 5.8, 95% CI 1.2 to 27.1) but not in hypertensives.[174] Hypertension did not modify the association between homocysteine and carotid intima-media thickness in our data.

In our study, distension was not associated with homocysteine, B vitamins or the MTHFR C677T polymorphism nor was distension related to many other study variables. The reliability of the duplicate distension measurements was high (r≅0.8) and difference between sonographers was low (0.02 mm). Although our results agree with de Bree and Lambert,[85,87] we suspected that elevated homocysteine and low folate would be associated with arterial stiffness based on human and animal studies. Biopsies from femoral arteries in hyperhomocysteinemic compared with normohomocysteinemic patients with occlusive peripheral vascular disease had a reduced smooth muscle cell/extracellular matrix ratio, which suggests that hyperhomocysteinemia is paired with greater arterial stiffness.[221] Rats on a folate-deplete diet compared with controls had lower carotid distension,[246] however folic acid supplementation did not affect markers of arterial stiffness in hyperhomocysteinemic mini-pigs.[233] Other animal models have shown an inverse association between homocysteine and measures of arterial stiffness.[247,248] In patients with end-stage renal disease, one-year supplementation with folic acid did not improve carotid distensibility.[91]

Is a ~0.05 mm greater carotid intima-media thickness associated with low folate concentrations of clinical significance? It resembles a five-year difference in age, given that carotid intima-media thickness progresses approximately 0.01 mm per year.[249] Furthermore, data from a similar Dutch population as our own has shown that for every 0.16 mm increase in carotid intima-media thickness, risk of myocardial infarction and risk of stroke increased by 50% and by 40%, respectively.[250] In our data, maximum carotid intima-media thickness was more often associated with the biochemical variables than mean carotid intima-media thickness, although both carotid intima-media thickness measurements were highly correlated. It is plausible that maximum carotid intima-media thickness more accurately captures the severity of atherosclerosis, considering that atherosclerotic changes are focal rather than diffuse.

Carotid intima-media thickness has been responsive to B vitamin intervention in vascular disease patients with carotid intima-media thickness ≥1 mm. Daily supplementation with folic acid, vitamin B_{12} and vitamin B_6 for one year led to carotid intima-media thickness regression by 4.2±12.8% whereas in the placebo group carotid intima-media thickness increased by 7.4±19.2%.[54] Similar findings have also been reported in renal transplant recipients with hyperhomocysteinemia.[55]

The greater risk of vascular disease morbidity and mortality associated with low concentrations of folate and increased homocysteine may originate from possible pathogenic effects on the coagulation or inflammation systems. We have shown that the association between folate deficiency and increased carotid intima-media thickness was independent of C-reactive protein. In the first 276 participants enrolled in FACIT, we have shown that C-reactive protein, fibrinogen and hemostasis markers did not respond to one-year folic acid supplementation (0.8 mg/d).[109]

Our findings support a pathogenic role of low folate, independent of homocysteine concentrations, in atherosclerosis. Clinical trials have already shown that carotid intima-media thickness quickly responds to B vitamin treatment in patient populations. Whether B vitamins decrease risk of vascular disease is currently under investigation.[236]

Chapter 4

High erythrocyte folate and the 5,10-methylenetetrahydrofolate reductase 677C→T mutation are associated with better cognitive performance

Jane Durga, Martin P.J. van Boxtel, Evert G. Schouten,
Michiel L. Bots, Frans J. Kok, Petra Verhoef

Division of Human Nutrition, Wageningen University, Wageningen, The Netherlands
Wageningen Centre for Food Sciences, Wageningen, The Netherlands
Department of Psychiatry and Neuropsychology, Brain and Behavior Institute,
Maastricht University, Maastricht, The Netherlands
Julius Center for Health Sciences and Primary Care, University Medical Center Utrecht,
Utrecht, The Netherlands

Submitted

Abstract

Background Low folate status has been associated with cognitive decline.

Aim We investigated the association of folate status and the 5,10-methylene-tetrahydrofolate reductase (MTHFR) 677C→T polymorphism with performance on a battery of neuropsychological tests. Furthermore, we investigated whether the association of folate with cognitive performance was mediated by plasma homocysteine or risk of vascular disease.

Methods We used cross-sectional data from 818 individuals aged 50 to 70 years old.

Results Low concentrations of erythrocyte folate but not serum folate were associated with poor performance on complex speed and memory tasks, independent of educational level and conventional risk factors of vascular disease. These associations were not mediated by homocysteine concentrations or carotid intima-media thickness. Subjects with the MTHFR 677TT genotype tended to perform better on cognitive tasks than CC/CT subjects, although this was significant for sensorimotor speed only (differences in *Z*-scores between MTHFR 677TT homozygotes and CC homozygotes -0.15, 95% CI -0.30 to 0.00).

Conclusion Low concentrations of erythrocyte folate are associated with decreased cognitive performance, possibly through a homocysteine-independent mechanism such as DNA infidelity and mitochondrial decay.

Introduction

Many individuals experience a decline in cognitive abilities as they grow older. In order to slow down or prevent this kind of cognitive decline, one needs to understand the factors that explain differences in the rate of cognitive decline with age between people. Nutritional factors that decrease with increasing age, like decreasing B vitamin concentrations, may help explain these variations.[93]

The B vitamins, specifically folate, have been implicated in neurological disorders, including those associated with cognitive disorders. Consumption of a folate-deplete diet for three months was associated with forgetfulness, paranoia and irritability.[251] These symptoms resided once folate in the diet was replenished. Likewise, in patients with deficient B vitamin levels or inborn errors of one-carbon metabolism, folate supplementation improved cognitive function.[252-259] Evidence from trials on the effect of folic acid supplementation on cognitive function in the general population is still inconclusive.[94] Many trials employed small study populations, lacked a control group or placebo treatment, allocated multiple interventions such that the effect of folate can not be delineated or employed rather insensitive tests, like the Mini-Mental Screening Examination.[47,95-100]

Several mechanisms may explain an association between folate and cognitive function. Recent evidence suggests that folate has antioxidant workings[108] and 10-formyltetrahydrofolate may help retain mitochondrial bioenergetic efficiency.[260] Low levels of folate have been speculated to impair methionine biosynthesis and *S*-adenosylmethionine production, thereby limiting methylation capacity.[92] Indeed, increased oxidative stress, mitochondrial bioenergetic inefficiency and hypomethylation have been linked to the aging and diseased brain.[261] The association between folate and cognitive performance may also be explained by increased concentrations of plasma homocysteine, a possible neurotoxic substance.[262-265] Both low folate concentrations and elevated homocysteine concentrations have been associated with increased risk of vascular disease,[32,36] which in turn has been implicated in decreased cognitive performance.[266-269] Whether the link between vascular disease and decreased cognitive function is explained by low concentrations of folate is unclear.

The common 5,10-methylenetetrahydrofolate reductase 677C→T polymorphism may give insight into the relation between folate and cognitive performance. The MTHFR 677TT genotype is associated with a decrease in MTHFR activity *in vitro* compared with the wild type enzyme.[202] MTHFR 677TT homozygotes compared with CC homozygotes are thought to have a higher formyl : methyl tetrahydrofolate derivative ratio,[207] hence a lower methylation capacity as indicated by elevated concentrations of homocysteine. Conversely, higher 10-formyltetrahydrofolate concentrations may salvage mitochondrial bioenergetic efficiency[260] and prevent cytotoxicity[270] and apoptosis.[271] Few studies have reported on the nature of the association of MTHFR C677T polymorphism with cognitive function. These studies were small and did not detect an association of MTHFR C677T polymorphism with high intelligence in children[272,273] or in older adults.[273]

In this study we examine the association of folate status with cognitive performance on a battery of tests probing different neuropsychological domains that tend to decline with age. We investigated whether the association between folate status and cognitive performance was mediated by homocysteine or risk of vascular disease, as measured by carotid intima-media thickness and carotid distension. Finally, we examined the relationship between MTHFR C677T polymorphism and cognitive performance.

Methods

Subjects

Data come from 819 men and post-menopausal women aged 50 to 70 years participating in the Folic Acid and Carotid Intima-media Thickness (FACIT) study, a single-center double blind randomized control trial investigating whether folic acid supplementation reduces the risk of cardiovascular disease, as measured by carotid intima-media thickness. Major exclusion criteria were homocysteine <13 μmol/L, vitamin B_{12} <200 pmol/L, renal or thyroid diseases and use of B vitamin supplements or medications that influence folate metabolism or atherosclerotic progression (e.g. lipid-lowering and hormone replacement therapies). The Medical Ethics Committee of Wageningen University approved the study and subjects gave written informed consent.

Cognitive function

Cognitive function was assessed using five separate tests: the Word Learning test, the Concept Shifting test, the Stroop Color-Word test, Verbal Fluency test and the Letter Digit Substitution test. The *Word Learning task* measures the storage and retrieval of newly acquired verbal material. Fifteen monosyllabic words are visually presented in a sequence, for two seconds each. The subjects are asked to recall the words immediately after each of the 3 presentation trials (immediate recall). Twenty minutes after the last trial, subjects are again prompted to recall the words (delayed recall). The number of correctly repeated words per trial is recorded. The *Concept Shifting task* estimates the ease of switching between two psychological concepts, as an index of perceptual planning and evaluation. First subjects are asked to cross out empty circles, then circles with numbers in chronological order and finally circles with letters in alphabetical order, randomly arranged in a circle. The final task is to alternately cross out circles with either numbers or letters, in chronological and alphabetical order. The time needed to complete the tasks is recorded. The *Stroop Color-Word test* measures selective attention and susceptibility to behavioral interference. Subjects are initially asked to read the name of colors (red, blue, green, yellow) and then name color blocks. Finally, subjects are asked to name the color of the ink rather than the word. The time needed to complete the tasks is recorded. The *Verbal Fluency test* measures the ability to draw on one's encyclopedic memory in a strategy-based manner. The subject is asked to name as many animals as possible in one minute. The number of different animals named is recorded. The *Letter Digit Substitution test* assesses general speed of visual information processing. Nine different letters are coupled with nine different numbers in a key on the top of the form. The subject is asked to copy the corresponding letter by each number as quickly as they can. The number of correctly filled in letters in ninety seconds is recorded. These tests were derived from the assessment protocol of the Maastricht Aging Study, a prospective study of the determinants of cognitive aging; for more extensive descriptions of these tests see Jolles et al.[274]

We included the Mini-Mental State Examination,[275] a widely used dementia-screening tool, to allow for comparison of our study population with other study populations and to exclude unreliable tests scores from subjects with suspected severe cognitive dysfunction (defined as <24 out of 30 points). All participants underwent the measurements after an overnight fast broken by a small snack consisting of a glass of juice and breakfast muffin. Trained research assistants administered the test during a 40-minute session to all but one participant; he was excluded from the data analyses.

Blood measurements

Fasting venous blood was collected, directly processed and stored at -80°C. Folate and vitamin B_{12} were measured using a chemiluminescent immunoassay (Immulite® 2000, Diagnostic Products Corporation). Erythrocyte folate was determined in duplicate and the average was taken to reduce measurement error. Serum creatinine and lipids were determined using Hitachi® 747 (Roche). We defined hypercholesterolemia as total cholesterol >6.5 mmol/L, high-density lipoprotein cholesterol (HDL) <0.9 mmol/L or use of lipid-lowering medication. Homocysteine was determined with HPLC and fluorimetric detection.[242] Vitamin B_6 was measured by HPLC. The C677T MTHFR genotype was determined by polymerase chain reaction of DNA and restriction enzyme digestion with *Hin*Fl. Intra-assay and inter-assay variation coefficients for laboratory analyses were <15%.

Carotid ultrasound

Carotid intima-media thickness, a valid surrogate marker of vascular disease and a structural marker of atherosclerosis[239] was measured using high-resolution B-mode sonography with a 7.5 MHz linear-array transducer (ATL UltraMark IX) as described earlier.[183] Longitudinal images of the distal common carotid arteries were frozen on the top of the R-wave. The mean of the maximum distances of the near and far wall of the distal 10 mm of the right and left common carotid artery was determined using an automated edge detection program. Carotid distension, a marker of arterial stiffness believed to increase as a result of aging and atherosclerosis,[240] was measured using M-mode sonography. The relative distension of the carotid artery was calculated as the absolute change in lumen diameter relative to its end-diastolic diameter was calculated. Ultrasound examination was performed in duplicate within three weeks; the average was used for analyses. The mean difference (± standard deviation [SD]) between the sonographers was 0.09 mm (±0.10 mm) for maximum intima-media thickness and 0.02 mm (±0.03 mm) for distension. The intraclass correlation coefficient for maximum intima-media thickness was 0.90 for sonographer 1 and 0.88 for sonographer 2 and for distension was 0.77 for sonographer 1 and 0.88 for sonographer 2.

Other measurements

A self-reported medical history, including current drug use and family history of premature vascular disease (onset <60 years in first degree family) and smoking were attained by questionnaire and reviewed by a research assistant. A participant was considered to have prevalent vascular disease if he had been clinically diagnosed with angina pectoris, myocardial infarction, arrhythmia, stroke, or peripheral arterial disease or if he had undergone certain palliative procedures (balloon angioplasty, coronary bypass surgery or aortic aneurysm surgery). Education was classified according the Dutch Central Bureau of Statistics and grouped according to highest attained level: primary education, junior vocational training or senior vocational/academic training. Height and weight were measured and body mass index (kg/m^2) was calculated. Blood pressure was measured using an automated meter (Dinamap® Compact Pro 100, General Electric) in supine position, while the participant underwent the ultrasound examination. The average of eight measurements was taken. We defined hypertension as systolic blood pressure ≥160 mmHg, diastolic blood pressure ≥95 mmHg or use of anti-hypertensive medication. Mean arterial pressure was calculated by the following formula: diastolic blood pressure + 1/3 · (systolic blood pressure – diastolic blood pressure). A food frequency questionnaire estimated folate intake and alcohol intake in the past three months. Two typists, blinded to study information, separately entered all data.

Statistical analysis

The domains—sensorimotor speed, complex speed and memory—were constructed by combining the results of Concept Shifting test, Stroop Color-Word test and Word learning test. In order to combine sub-tests, *Z*-scores were calculated. Sensorimotor speed index is a measure for basic speed and is compromised of the first two trials in the Concept Shifting test and Stroop Color-Word test, whereas complex speed index, a measure of cognitive flexibility and the ability to switch between different tasks, is composed of the final trials of the same tests. The verbal memory index is calculated using the total and the maximum of the three immediate recall trials and the delayed recall score. See van Boxtel et al for an extensive description of this data reduction method.[101] The Letter Digit Substitution test and Verbal Fluency test were not included in compound measures, however, for ease of comparison we converted the raw scores to *Z*-scores as well.

For each participant, we averaged the homocysteine concentrations measured at screening and at baseline and used this average in the analyses. To investigate the association between folate and cognitive performance, the mean adjusted cognitive performance was calculated based on folate status: deficiency (erythrocyte folate ≤305 nmol/L; serum folate ≤7 nmol/L), low-normal (erythrocyte folate 306-500 nmol/L; serum folate 8-11 nmol/L) and high-normal (erythrocyte folate ≥501 nmol/L; serum folate ≥12 nmol/L). Adjustment was done initially for age, sex and education level and then for other possible confounders. Possible confounders were hypertension, total cholesterol, HDL, hypercholesterolemia, serum creatinine, apoE ε4 allele, diabetes mellitus, body mass index, current smoking, smoking pack years and alcohol intake. To examine whether the association between folate and cognitive performance may be mediated by homocysteine or vascular disease risk, we included homocysteine or carotid intima-media thickness or carotid distension. We included mean arterial pressure as a covariate in the analyses involving distension. Because the MTHFR 677T allele is associated with hyperhomocysteinemia mainly when folate concentrations are low,[39] we stratified the population based on folate status and studied the relationship between genotype and cognitive performance levels within these strata. The latter analyses were adjusted for age, sex and education level using analysis of covariance. Statistical significance was defined as $p<0.05$ (two-tailed). Statistical analyses were performed using SPSS 11.0 for Windows.

Results

Table 4.1 shows the characteristics of the study population. Nine percent, 2% and 13% of the participants had deficient levels of serum folate, erythrocyte folate and vitamin B_6 according to the American Institute of Medicine.[245] The MTHFR 677T allelic distribution did not significantly differ from the calculated expected distribution, assuming a Hardy-Weinberg equilibrium. Table 4.2 shows the raw scores of the individual tests before Z-scores were calculated. Seven subjects scored <24 points out of 30 on the Mini-mental state examination, which may indicate a cognitive disorder. The associations of folate status and MTHFR 677TT genotype with cognitive performance were similar regardless if these subjects were excluded from the analyses, thus we presented the results from the total population. Second to educational level, age was a strong determinant of performance on cognitive tests. The association with age was greater for complex speed and information processing and weakest for Verbal Fluency test, after adjustment for conventional risk factors of vascular disease (sensorimotor speed $\beta=-0.038$ (standard error 0.005), $p<0.001$; complex speed $\beta=-0.040$ (0.005), $p<0.001$; memory $\beta=-0.029$ (0.006), $p<0.001$; Letter Digit Substitution test $\beta=-0.043$ (0.006), $p<0.001$; Verbal Fluency $\beta=-0.018$ (0.006), $p=0.005$).

Folate and cognitive performance

Subjects with serum folate deficiency performed on average poorer on the Verbal Fluency test than subjects with low-normal and high-normal concentrations of serum folate (mean difference in Z-scores between deficient vs. high-normal concentrations -0.29, 95% CI -0.54 to -0.04). The difference between the groups weakened when age, sex and educational level were entered into the regression model (mean difference in Z-scores between deficient vs. high-normal concentrations -0.25, 95% CI -0.49 to -0.01) and became non-significant when conventional risk factors for vascular disease were entered into the regression model (mean difference in Z-scores between deficient vs.

Table 4.1 Population characteristics (*n*=818).

		Mean (standard deviation) Median (interquartile range)
Demographics		
	Age, years	60 ± 6
	% Male	72
	% Low / Middle / High education level	22 / 38 / 40
Markers of vascular disease		
	Maximum carotid intima-media thickness, mm	1.02 ± 0.17
	Carotid distension, mm	0.63 ± 0.17
	% Familial history of premature vascular disease	21
	% Vascular disease	12
Clinical		
	Homocysteine, μmol/L	13.8 ± 2.3
	% 5,10-methyenetetrahydrofolate reductase 677 CC / CT / TT	38 / 46 / 15
	Serum folate, nmol/L	12 ± 4
	Erythrocyte folate, nmol/L	697 ± 267
	Vitamin B_{12}, pmol/L	296 (250 to 376)
	Vitamin B_6, nmol/L	35 ± 20
	Body mass index, kg/m^2	26 ± 4
	Creatinine, μmol/L	93 ± 12
	High-density lipoprotein cholesterol, mmol/L	1.2 ± 0.4
	Total cholesterol, mmol/L	5.8 ± 1.1
	% Hypercholesterolemia	36
	Systolic BP, mmHg	133 ± 16
	Diastolic BP, mmHg	77 ± 8
	% Hypertension	22
	% Diabetes mellitus	3
	% apoE ε4 allele, 0 / 1 / 2	68 / 29 / 3
Lifestyle		
	% Current smokers	20
	Folate intake, μg/d	207 ± 77
	Alcohol intake, g/d	13 (4 to 23)

high-normal concentrations -0.22, 95% CI -0.47 to 0.02). Serum folate concentrations were not associated with the other domains.

Erythrocyte folate deficiency, on the other hand, was associated with poor performance on a variety of cognitive tests despite the small number of individuals with deficient erythrocyte folate concentrations. In crude analyses, subjects with deficient concentrations of erythrocyte folate performed poorer on all cognitive tests than

Table 4.2 Performance on cognitive function tests.

	n	Mean (standard deviation) Median (interquartile range)
Mini-Mental State Examination, points	818	29 (28 to 30)
<24 out of 30 points	7	
Verbal Fluency test, words	818	24 ± 6
15 Word Learning test	818	
Total of 3 trials, words		27 ± 6
Maximum of 3 trials, words		11 ± 2
Delayed recall, words		9 ± 3
Letter Digit Substitution test, digits in 90 s	815	49 ± 9
Concept Shifting test		
Empty, s	817	5 ± 1
Numbers, s	818	22 (19 to 26)
Letters, s	814	25 (22 to 30)
Numbers and letters, s	814	36 ± 13
Stroop Color-Word test		
Reading name of colors, s	817	16 ± 3
Naming color of ink, s	815	43 ± 11

subjects with high-normal concentrations, however, this did not reach statistical significance for the Verbal Fluency test. After adjustment for age, sex and educational level, the associations remained for sensorimotor speed, complex speed and memory (mean difference in *Z*-scores between deficient vs. high-normal concentrations: sensorimotor speed -0.33, 95% CI -0.65 to -0.01; complex speed -0.52, 95% CI -0.88 to -0.16; memory -0.52, -0.92 to -0.11). The association of erythrocyte folate with cognitive performance remained statistically significant for complex speed and memory after adjustment for conventional risk factors of vascular disease (mean difference in *Z*-scores between deficient vs. high-normal concentrations: sensorimotor speed -0.27, 95% CI -0.60 to 0.07; complex speed -0.45, 95% CI -0.82 to -0.08; memory -0.50, 95% CI -0.92 to -0.10) (Figure 4.1).

We examined whether the association between deficient concentrations of erythrocyte folate and cognitive performance might be mediated by elevated concentrations of homocysteine or increased risk of vascular disease, the latter estimated by increased intima-media thickness or low distension. Age and sex adjusted erythrocyte folate concentrations were correlated with homocysteine concentrations (r=-0.26, p<0.001) and with intima-media thickness (r=-0.08, p=0.019), but not with distension. In addition, homocysteine concentrations were correlated with sensorimotor and complex speed (partial correlation coefficient: sensorimotor speed r=-0.07, p=0.040; complex speed r= -0.07, p=0.049) and intima-media thickness was correlated with sensorimotor and complex speed and the Letter Digit Substitution test (partial correlation coefficient: sensorimotor speed r=-0.09, p=0.017; complex speed r=-0.09, p=0.014; Letter Digit Substitution test r=-0.06, p=0.083) independent of conventional risk factors for vascular disease. Addition of variables on vascular disease prevalence or familial history of premature vascular disease did not significantly affect the association of intima-media thickness and cognitive performance. The association between erythrocyte folate and complex speed was independent of homocysteine concentrations (mean difference deficient vs. high-normal concentrations: complex speed -0.39, 95% CI -0.76 to -0.01) and independent of intima-media thickness or other markers of vascular disease (i.e., vascular disease prevalence and familial history of premature vascular disease) (mean difference in Z-scores between deficient vs. high-normal concentrations: complex speed -0.44, 95% CI -0.80 to -0.07).

MTHFR and cognitive function

Despite similar folate intake, subjects with the MTHFR 677TT genotype had higher homocysteine concentrations and lower serum folate concentrations than CC or CT subjects (homocysteine 15.3 vs. 14.2 μmol/L, p<0.001; serum folate 11 vs. 13 nmol/L, p=0.001). No other study variables differed between the MTHFR C677T genotypes. MTHFR 677TT homozygotes tended to have higher cognitive performance scores on all tests except Verbal Fluency than CC homozygotes, with CT heterozygotes having intermediate values (Figure 4.2). In subjects with a folate status below that of the population median, having the MTHFR 677TT genotype was often associated with better performance on sensorimotor and complex speed (Table 4.3). Folate intake, in contrast to blood concentrations of folate, was not likely to be influenced by MTHFR C677T genotype. When the population was stratified on the basis of folate intake, MTHFR 677TT homozygotes in the upper half of the folate intake distribution tended to show better cognitive performance compared with their CC or CT counterparts. Folate intake was weakly correlated with blood folate levels (erythrocyte folate r=0.11, p=0.002; serum folate r=0.16, p<0.001, adjusted for age, sex and MTHFR C677T genotype).

Table 4.3 Mean performance (*Z*-score) on cognitive tests per 5,10-methylenetetrahydrofolate reductase (MTHFR) 677C→T genotype, adjusted for age, sex and educational level.

	Mean (95% confidence interval)						P_{trend}
MTHFR C677T genotype	CC		CT		TT		
Serum folate[a]							
<50 percentile							
Sensorimotor speed	-0.08	(-0.21 to 0.04)	-0.08	(-0.18 to 0.03)	0.13	(-0.04 to 0.30)	0.078
Complex speed	-0.10	(-0.24 to 0.04)	-0.05	(-0.17 to 0.07)	0.12	(-0.07 to 0.31)	0.079
Memory	-0.11	(-0.26 to 0.04)	0.00	(-0.13 to 0.12)	-0.01	(-0.21 to 0.19)	0.359
Letter digit substitution	-0.05	(-0.20 to 0.11)	-0.03	(-0.16 to 0.11)	0.03	(-0.18 to 0.24)	0.574
Verbal fluency	-0.02	(-0.18 to 0.15)	-0.12	(-0.27 to 0.02)	0.02	(-0.21 to 0.25)	0.489
>50 percentile							
Sensorimotor speed	0.00	(-0.10 to 0.10)	0.05	(-0.04 to 0.15)	0.07	(-0.12 to 0.25)	0.460
Complex speed	0.05	(-0.05 to 0.16)	0.04	(-0.06 to 0.14)	0.02	(-0.18 to 0.22)	0.744
Memory	0.05	(-0.09 to 0.18)	-0.02	(-0.14 to 0.11)	0.21	(-0.03 to 0.46)	0.546
Letter digit substitution	0.01	(-0.13 to 0.15)	0.00	(-0.13 to 0.13)	0.15	(-0.10 to 0.41)	0.484
Verbal fluency	0.04	(-0.10 to 0.18)	0.09	(-0.04 to 0.23)	0.02	(-0.24 to 0.29)	0.817
Erythrocyte folate[b]							
<50 percentile							
Sensorimotor speed	-0.18	(-0.30 to -0.05)	-0.10	(-0.20 to -0.03)	0.08	(-0.10 to 0.27)	0.031
Complex speed	-0.16	(-0.31 to -0.02)	-0.06	(-0.18 to 0.05)	0.11	(-0.10 to 0.33)	0.041
Memory	0.03	(-0.12 to 0.18)	-0.03	(-0.15 to 0.09)	0.05	(-0.18 to 0.28)	0.958
Letter digit substitution	-0.13	(-0.29 to 0.03)	-0.09	(-0.22 to 0.04)	-0.01	(-0.26 to 0.23)	0.446
Verbal fluency	-0.10	(-0.27 to 0.06)	-0.07	(-0.20 to 0.05)	0.09	(-0.16 to 0.34)	0.452
>50 percentile							
Sensorimotor speed	0.07	(-0.03 to 0.17)	0.09	(-0.01 to 0.20)	0.13	(-0.04 to 0.29)	0.578
Complex speed	0.10	(-0.08 to 0.20)	0.06	(-0.05 to 0.17)	0.06	(-0.11 to 0.23)	0.640
Memory	-0.06	(-0.19 to 0.07)	0.01	(-0.13 to 0.14)	0.11	(-0.10 to 0.32)	0.168
Letter digit substitution	0.07	(-0.06 to 0.20)	0.07	(-0.06 to 0.21)	0.16	(-0.05 to 0.38)	0.571
Verbal fluency	0.10	(-0.04 to 0.25)	0.04	(-0.10 to 0.20)	-0.02	(-0.27 to 0.21)	0.653

Table 4.3 (*Continued*).

	Mean (95% confidence interval)						P_{trend}
MTHFR C677T genotype	CC		CT		TT		
Folate intake[c]							
<50 percentile							
Sensorimotor speed	0.02	(-0.09 to 0.13)	-0.03	(-0.13 to 0.06)	0.07	(-0.11 to 0.24)	0.967
Complex speed	0.03	(-0.09 to 0.16)	0.04	(-0.07 to 0.14)	0.10	(-0.10 to 0.30)	0.665
Memory	-0.06	(-0.20 to 0.07)	0.06	(-0.06 to 0.18)	0.14	(-0.08 to 0.36)	0.091
Letter digit substitution	0.04	(-0.10 to 0.19)	0.08	(-0.04 to 0.21)	0.08	(-0.16 to 0.32)	0.732
Verbal fluency	0.09	(-0.07 to 0.25)	-0.01	(-0.15 to 0.12)	0.04	(-0.22 to 0.29)	0.615
>50 percentile							
Sensorimotor speed	-0.10	(-0.21 to 0.02)	0.02	(-0.09 to 0.13)	0.14	(-0.04 to 0.32)	0.021
Complex speed	-0.07	(-0.19 to 0.05)	-0.06	(-0.18 to 0.05)	0.09	(-0.10 to 0.27)	0.258
Memory	0.01	(-0.13 to 0.15)	-0.10	(-0.23 to 0.04)	0.04	(-0.18 to 0.25)	0.868
Letter digit substitution	-0.09	(-0.23 to 0.05)	-0.12	(-0.25 to 0.02)	0.09	(-0.13 to 0.30)	0.315
Verbal fluency	-0.07	(-0.22 to 0.08)	-0.10	(-0.16 to 0.14)	0.03	(-0.23 to 0.24)	0.807

[a] Median cut-off serum folate: 11.7 nmol/L; <50 percentile serum folate: *n*=143 CC, *n*=192 CT, *n*=76 TT; >50 percentile serum folate *n*=168 CC, *n*=186 CT, *n*=49 TT.

[b] Median cut-off erythrocyte folate 657 nmol/L; <50 percentile erythrocyte folate: *n*=132 CC, *n*=215 CT, *n*=59 TT; >50 percentile erythrocyte folate *n*=179 CC, *n*=163 CT, *n*=66 TT.

[c] Median cut-off folate intake 195 µg/d; <50 percentile folate intake: *n*=148 CC, *n*=203 CT, *n*=56 TT; >50 percentile folate intake *n*=163 CC, *n*=175 CT, *n*=69 TT.

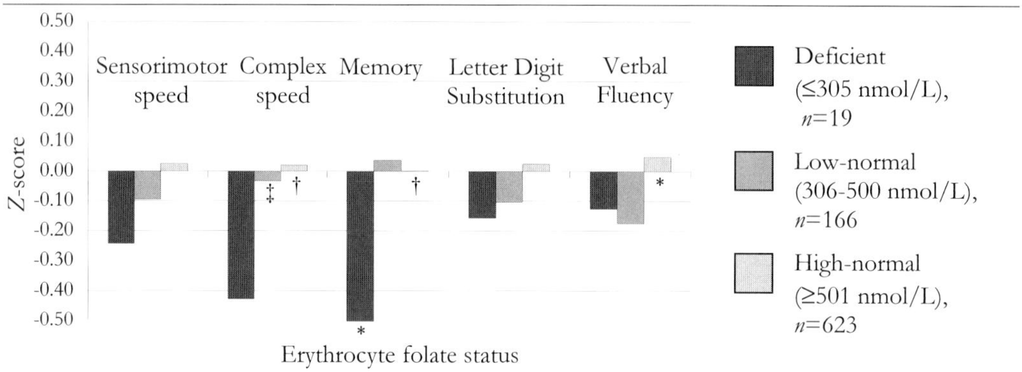

Figure 4.1 Mean performance (Z-score) on sensorimotor speed, complex speed and memory tasks by erythrocyte folate status, adjusted for age, sex, educational level and conventional risk factors of vascular disease.
* $p<0.01$ vs. low-normal.
† $p<0.02$ vs. deficient.
‡ $p=0.039$ vs. deficient.

Discussion

We have shown that deficient levels of erythrocyte folate were associated with poor cognitive domains, i.e. complex speed and memory, independent of risk factors for vascular disease, including homocysteine and intima-media thickness. Contrary to our expectations, subjects with the MTHFR 677TT genotype often performed better on cognitive tests, although this was statistically significant for sensorimotor speed only. When we examined the relation between MTHFR C677T polymorphism and cognitive performance stratified by folate status, having the MTHFR 677TT genotype was associated with better performance on sensorimotor and complex speed in individuals with a low folate status. Folate intake, unlike serum or erythrocyte folate concentrations, is unlikely to be influenced by the MTHFR C677T genotype and hence is more appropriate to examine effect modification due to folate. However, the positive association of MTHFR 677TT genotype and cognitive performance was strongest among those with high folate intake rather than low folate intake.

In our study deficient levels of erythrocyte folate were linked to poor performance on tests probing cognitive domains susceptible to age-related cognitive decline, like sensorimotor and complex speed and memory.[101] Some studies support a role of folate in memory processes. Studies in folate deficient individuals show increased 'forgetfulness' during folate depletion ($n=1$)[251] whereas supplementation was associated with improved memory scores after two months ($n=30$).[97] Unfortunately, these studies did not measure speed-related domains like sensorimotor or complex speed. We are unsure why the

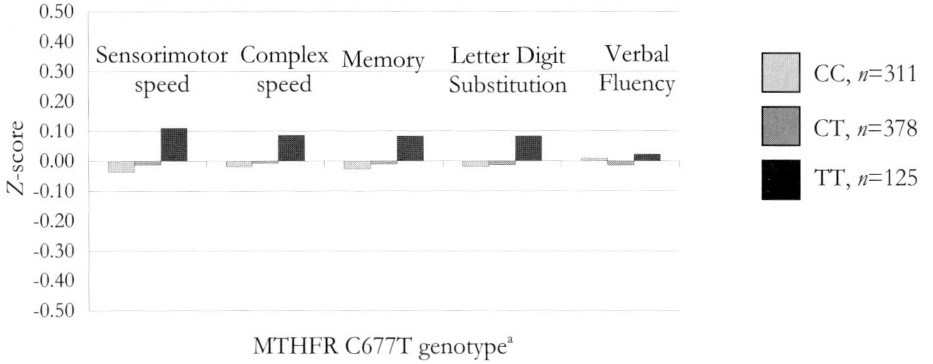

Figure 4.2 Mean performance of neuropsychological battery (Z-score) by 5,10-methylenetetrahydrofolate reductase (MTHFR) 677C→T genotype, adjusted for age, sex and educational level.

* $p<0.05$ vs. CC.

[a] CC n=310 and CT n=376 in Letter Digit Substitution test, respectively; CT n=377 in complex speed.

why the association between folate and cognitive performance was stronger with erythrocyte folate rather than with serum folate. The two measures were correlated (r=0.51, $p<0.001$) as would be expected: erythrocyte folate is conventionally considered a marker of long-term folate status whereas serum folate is considered a short-term dietary folate intake marker. Other studies conducted in the general population also have found inconsistencies in associations between the folate markers with cognitive performance.[276-278]

Due to the cross-sectional nature of our study we are unable to investigate whether low concentrations of folate are a cause of poor cognitive performance. Theoretically, the association between erythrocyte folate and cognitive function may be explained by reverse causality and the association may be confounded (low folate status is related to many 'unhealthy' lifestyles which cannot be completely controlled for by adjustment). Larger prospective and intervention studies are needed to determine whether low folate status is implicated in age-related cognitive decline and whether folic acid supplementation or an increase in dietary folate can prevent or reverse age-related cognitive decline.

Examination of the association of MTHFR C677T genotype with performance on cognitive tests, however, transforms our cross-sectional study into a prospective study ('Mendelian randomization') and helps reduce bias and confounding associated with a dietary marker like blood folate concentrations, as the genotype is unlikely to affect other factors than folate metabolism ('Mendelian deconfounding').[76,279] The premise being that after conception and birth, individuals are 'randomly assigned' to their MTHFR C677T genotype, and depending on gene-environment interaction, also have lifelong exposure to their MTHFR C677T phenotype, such as homocysteine concentrations. Thus, genotype establishes lifelong risk (adequate induction period), cannot be changed by cognitive decline (no reverse causality) and probably is not linked to other environmental risk factors for cognitive decline (no or little confounding). In our population, MTHFR 677TT homozygosity was paired with better cognitive performance on all tests, except Verbal Fluency; however, this was statistically significant for sensorimotor speed only. When folate status is low, phenotypic expression of the MTHFR 677TT genotype is most pronounced, i.e. concentrations of homocysteine increase. An elevated concentration of homocysteine, a putative independent risk factor for reduced sensorimotor and complex speed in our data but also confirmed by other investigators, is the conventional consequence of MTHFR 677TT phenotype, however other changes have been documented in folate/one-carbon metabolism which may help explain the protective effect of MTHFR 677TT genotype.

A possible protective effect of the MTHFR 677TT genotype may lie in its greater relative one-carbon commitment to *de novo* synthesis of nucleotides and an increase in formyl-folate derivatives relative to methyl-folate derivatives. In theory, subjects with a greater capacity of thymidylate synthesis and 10-formyltetrahydrofolate generation may have a reduced risk of genomic and mitochondrial DNA damage in two ways. Individuals with the MTHFR 677TT genotype may have increased thymidylate synthesis that may directly reduce DNA mutations by ensuring a smaller pool of uracil. Secondly, MTHFR 677TT homozygotes may have greater amounts of 10-formyltetrahydrofolate that may protect mitochondrial integrity by reducing cytochrome *c* [260] and may have other antioxidant-like functions in the cytosol and mitochondria.

Conversely, our genetic data do not support the hypomethylation theory of cognitive decline[92,93] brought forth by Osmond and Smythies in 1952.[280] In support of the hypomethylation theory, studies have shown lower concentrations of *S*-adenosylmethionine and DNA hypomethylation in the brain of MTHFR-heterozygotes knockout mice compared with wild type.[281] In humans, supplementation with methyl donors (e.g. betaine and *S*-adenosylmethionine) alleviates neurological symptoms in patients with low or undetectable levels of MTHFR activity[282] and may improve cognitive performance in subjects with cognitive deficits without affecting total folate concentrations.[283] Theoretically, however, supplementation with *S*-adenosylmethionine (an allosteric inhibitor of MTHFR) may shift the distribution of folate derivatives in favor of formyl-folates at the expense of methyl-folates, mimicking to some extent the MTHFR 677TT genotype.

The major limitation of this study is that it may be underpowered to find gene-disease marker associations. Thus, better cognitive performance among those with the MTHFR 677TT genotype may be a chance finding. Furthermore, the homocysteine inclusion criterion may have biased our results. This has surely increased the number of subjects with the MTHFR 677TT genotype in our study (~15% in our study vs. ~10% in the general Dutch population),[39] but since both MTHFR 677TT genotype and lifestyle factors, e.g. smoking and low fruit and vegetable intake, influence homocysteine concentrations, we may have inadvertently selected 'healthy' MTHFR 677TT homozygotes, and compared them with their more 'unhealthy' CC and CT counterparts. However, all of the risk factors presented in Table 4.1 were not statistically different between the genotype groups, except for serum folate and homocysteine concentrations. Furthermore, addition of conventional risk factors to the analyses investigating the relationship between genotype and cognitive function did not affect the association. On the other hand, our study population was not exposed to folic acid fortification nor reported use of B vitamin supplements; thus an association between MTHFR 677TT genotype and cognitive function may be easier to detect compared with studies conducted in populations with folic acid fortification.

Despite our efforts to limit the number of dependent variables by combining relevant raw test scores into a compound performance index, in this study several independent null hypotheses were tested. Therefore, one should be cautious with interpretation of the results, considering that the study was relatively large and the association estimates relatively small. Furthermore, from this cross-sectional analysis, it is not possible to determine whether low levels of folate precede poor cognitive performance. Low intake of folate may be a consequence of cognitive decline, i.e. agnosia and apraxia may lead to a decrease in folate intake.[284] Furthermore, amnesia may differentially affect the accuracy of dietary intake recall. Thus, it is important to conduct randomized controlled trials using a battery of tests sensitive to cognitive decline associated with aging. We will evaluate the three-year effect of supplementation with folic acid versus placebo on cognitive tests described in this study and shall report in 2005. Furthermore, larger observational studies and meta-analysis of observational studies investigating the association of common mutations in folate-related genes with cognitive function are needed to understand the possible etiology of folate-related cognitive decline and dementia.

Chapter 5

Association of serum folate with hearing is dependent on the 5,10-methylenetetrahdyrofolate reductase 677C→T mutation

Jane Durga, Lucien J.C. Anteunis, Evert G. Schouten,
Michiel L. Bots, Frans J. Kok, Petra Verhoef

Division of Human Nutrition, Wageningen University, Wageningen, The Netherlands
Wageningen Centre for Food Sciences, Wageningen, The Netherlands
Division of Audiology, Brain and Behavior Institute, University Hospital Maastricht, Maastricht, The Netherlands
Julius Center for Health Sciences and Primary Care, University Medical Center Utrecht, Utrecht, The Netherlands

Submitted

Abstract

Background Vascular disease and its risk factors may explain variation in age-related hearing loss.

Aim We examined the association of elevated plasma homocysteine and its determinants—low B vitamin concentrations and the 5,10-methylenetetrahydrofolate reductase (MTHFR) 677C→T polymorphism—with hearing levels.

Methods We used cross-sectional data from 729 individuals with sensorineural hearing loss. Hearing was assessed as the average of the pure-tone air conduction thresholds for both ears for 0.5 kHz, 1 kHz and 2 kHz and for 4 kHz, 6 kHz and 8 kHz.

Results Homocysteine, erythrocyte folate and vitamin B_6 were not associated with hearing thresholds. Low concentrations of serum folate and vitamin B_{12} were associated with better hearing, independent of vascular disease risk factors. MTHFR 677TT homozygotes had similar hearing levels as subjects with a C allele when folate status was below the median. However, when folate status was above population median, MTHFR 677TT homozygotes had on average ~5 dB (p=0.027) lower hearing thresholds than subjects with a 677C allele. The relationship between serum folate and hearing thresholds appeared to be dependent on MTHFR C677T genotype (CC r=0.12 p=0.033; TT r=-0.12 p=0.187).

Conclusion Our findings due not support an association of elevated homocysteine with hearing impairment, but rather support the hypothesis that a greater one-carbon moiety commitment to *de novo* synthesis is protective for hearing.

Introduction

Age-related hearing loss is one of the most prevalent chronic conditions affecting the elderly. Age-related hearing loss is a bilateral sensorineural hearing loss initially affecting the higher frequencies and subsequently extending towards the lower frequencies. Decline in hearing acuity may begin in the third and fourth decade of life, although it is not inevitable.[285] Age accounts for 10% of the variation in age-related hearing loss,[286] thus factors that vary with age may play an etiological role in age-related hearing loss. Age-related changes in vascular and neural tissue of the cochlea are thought to contribute to age-related hearing loss. These neural and vascular changes in the cochlea may be secondary to mitochondrial dysfunction.[287,288]

More than 100 years ago investigators contemplated the relation between arteriosclerosis in cochlear arterial beds and arteriosclerosis in other vascular beds in the body[289,290] (references therein). From histopathological studies of the cochleae of elderly subjects, arteriosclerosis in the inner ear has been associated with decreased hearing levels and with atherosclerosis in the coronary and renal arteries.[290] It wasn't until the seminal work of Rosen and coworkers on the Mabaan tribe in Sudan, however, that much epidemiologic research on the relation of vascular disease and vascular disease risk factors with age-related hearing loss was generated.[285] Although the majority of studies demonstrate an association of vascular disease with hearing levels,[291-297] the association of vascular disease risk factors, like smoking, hypertension, hypercholesterolemia, with hearing levels has been inconsistent.[290,295,298-303]

Recently, Berner and colleagues examined the association between hearing levels and plasma total homocysteine, a novel risk factor for vascular disease.[103] Homocysteine was only marginally associated with hearing levels in 91 audiological patients. To our knowledge no studies have examined the effects associated with elevated concentrations of homocysteine on cochlear tissue, nevertheless, possible mechanisms can be extrapolated from vascular disease research. Elevated concentrations of homocysteine have been associated with smooth muscle cell proliferation[226] and changes in microvessel flow mechanics.[248,304] These changes may be linked to changes in microvessel permeability,[248] cochlear blood flow and stria vascularis atrophy. Apart from atherogenic properties, homocysteine is considered to have neurotoxic properties, as well, which may adversely influence the highly innervated cochlea. For example, homocysteine may act as an agonist at the glutamate site of the N-methyl-D-aspartate receptor.[305] Poor hearing has been associated with over excitation of N-methyl-D-aspartate receptors.[306]

In contrast to the very weak association found between homocysteine and hearing levels,[103] determinants of elevated concentrations of homocysteine, such as low concentrations of folate and vitamin B_{12} have been inversely associated with hearing levels in women with age-related hearing loss.[102,103] However, Berner and colleagues reported a null association of folate and vitamin B_{12} with hearing levels.[103] No studies have examined the association of polymorphisms associated with elevated concentrations of homocysteine and hearing. Approximately 10% of the Dutch population has a cytosine-to-thymidine transition in the *methylenetetrahydrofolate reductase* (*MTHFR*) gene at nucleotide 677. This mutation results in an alanine-to-valine substitution in the MTHFR protein and leads to a decrease in MTHFR activity compared with the wild type enzyme.[202] Individuals with the MTHFR 677TT genotype tend to have higher concentrations of homocysteine, especially pronounced when folate concentrations are low.[307]

Determinants of elevated concentrations of homocysteine may also have direct effects on neural tissue and vascular tissue of the cochlea, independent of their association with homocysteine or vascular disease. Recent evidence suggests that folate has antioxidant-like properties[108,260,308] which may protect the cochlea from reactive oxygen species mediated damage. Finally, low concentrations of vitamins B_{12} and B_6 may also have neurotoxic effects. Animal studies have shown that deficiencies in vitamins B_{12} and B_6 have been associated with demyelinization of the auditory neurological tissue and other cochlear malformations.[309]

We hypothesize that an elevated concentration of homocysteine and its determinants—the MTHFR 677TT genotype and decreased concentrations of B vitamins—are associated with poor hearing. Furthermore, we examine whether the association of homocysteine and B vitamins with hearing levels remains after adjustment for vascular disease, including markers of atherosclerosis and arterial stiffness.

Methods

Subjects

Data are from 819 men and post-menopausal women aged 50 to 70 years participating in the Folic Acid and Carotid Intima-media Thickness (FACIT) study, a trial investigating whether folic acid supplementation can halt the progression of atherosclerosis. Major exclusion criteria were homocysteine <13 μmol/L, vitamin B_{12} <200 pmol/L, renal or thyroid diseases and use of B vitamin supplements or medications that influence folate metabolism or atherosclerotic progression (e.g. lipid-lowering and hormone replacement therapies). Ninety subjects were excluded because of hearing loss attributed to middle ear dysfunction (air-bone gap ≥15 dB in either ear) or unilateral hearing loss (a difference in average pure-tone hearing thresholds for 0.5 kHz, 1 kHz, 2 kHz ≥20 dB between the right and left ear). The Medical Ethics Committee of Wageningen University approved the study and subjects gave written informed consent.

Audiometric measurements

Subjects' ears were examined for excessive cerumen, which was removed if present. Pure-tone air and bone conduction thresholds were obtained with subjects seated in an acoustical booth (Audiofon G, Audiovox Italy) using a portable diagnostic audiometer (Voyager 522). We calculated average pure-tone air conduction thresholds of 0.5, 1 and 2 kHz (PTA-low) and of 4, 6 and 8 kHz (PTA-high). Audiometric testing was done using a variation of the Hughson and Westlake method: thresholds based on ascending responses using up 5 dB, down 10 dB steps.[310] Contralateral masking was used when necessary. Twenty-nine subjects had a hearing threshold at a number of frequencies that was not measurable by our audiometer (maximum pure-tone air conduction emitted was 100 dB; 2 kHz n=1, 4 kHz n=4, 6 kHz n=6, 8 kHz n=29). These subjects were assigned a hearing threshold of 105 dB, as it was assumed that their hearing threshold was greater than 100 dB.

Blood measurements

Fasting venous blood was collected, directly processed and stored at -80°C. Folate and vitamin B_{12} were measured using a chemiluminescent immunoassay (Immulite® 2000, Diagnostic Products Corporation). Erythrocyte folate was determined in duplicate and the average was taken to reduce measurement error. Serum creatinine and lipids were determined using Hitachi® 747 (Roche). We defined hypercholesterolemia as total cholesterol >6.5 mmol/L, high-density lipoprotein cholesterol <0.9 mmol/L or use of lipid-lowering medication. Homocysteine was determined with HPLC and fluorimetric detection.[242] Vitamin B_6 was measured by HPLC. The C677T MTHFR genotype was determined by polymerase chain reaction of DNA and restriction enzyme digestion with *Hin*Fl. Intra-assay and inter-assay variation coefficients for laboratory analyses were <15%.

Carotid ultrasound

Carotid intima-media thickness, a valid surrogate marker of vascular disease and a structural marker of atherosclerosis,[239] was measured using high-resolution B-mode ultrasonography with a 7.5 MHz linear-array transducer (ATL UltraMark IX). Longitudinal images of the distal common carotid arteries were obtained at four predefined angles of 30° steps (90° to 180° on the right side and 270° to 180° on the left side). Images were frozen on the top of the R-wave of the electrocardiography and recorded on VHS tape. The maximum distance of the near and far wall of the distal 10 mm of the right and left common carotid artery was determined using an automated edge detection program. Carotid distension, a marker of arterial stiffness believed to increase as a result of aging and atherosclerosis,[240,311] was measured using M-mode sonography. An M-line was placed at an angle deemed by the sonographer to give the best visualization of the arterial walls. The sonographer recorded carotid artery pulsation for approximately three seconds. The relative distension of the carotid artery was calculated as the absolute change in lumen diameter relative to its end-diastolic diameter was calculated. The average of three measurements per side was calculated. Ultrasound examinations were performed in duplicate within three weeks; the average was used for analyses. The intraclass correlation coefficient for intima-media thickness was 0.89 and for distension was 0.87. The same sonographer performed both examinations in 91% of the subjects. A single reader interpreted all images. Both sonographers and the reader were blinded to participants' study information.

Other measurements

A self-reported medical history, including current drug use and family history of premature vascular disease (onset <60 years in first degree family), and smoking were attained by questionnaire and reviewed by a research assistant. A participant was considered to have prevalent vascular disease if he had been diagnosed with angina pectoris, myocardial infarction, arrhythmia, stroke, or peripheral arterial disease or if he had undergone certain palliative procedures (balloon angioplasty, coronary bypass surgery or aortic aneurysm surgery). Height and weight were measured and body mass index (kg/m^2) was calculated. Blood pressure was measured using an automated meter (Dinamap® Compact Pro 100, General Electric) in supine position, while the participant underwent the ultrasound examination. The average of eight measurements was taken. We defined hypertension as systolic blood pressure ≥160 mmHg, diastolic blood pressure ≥95 mmHg or use of antihypertensive medication. Mean arterial pressure was calculated by the following formula: diastolic blood pressure + 1/3 · (systolic blood pressure – diastolic blood pressure). A food frequency questionnaire estimated folate intake and alcohol intake in the past three months. Two typists, blinded to study information, separately entered all data.

Statistical analysis

For each participant, we averaged the homocysteine and vitamin B_{12} concentrations measured at screening and at baseline and used this average in the analyses. The average of the right and left ear PTA hearing threshold was used for the analyses. After transformation (natural log) of the PTA-low and PTA-high distributions to obtain normality, the relation between conventional risk factors of vascular disease and (sub-clinical) markers of vascular disease and PTA-low and PTA-high were assessed using linear regression. In order to calculate mean hearing thresholds among tertiles of homocysteine and B vitamins, we employed analysis of covariance. Test for trend was extracted from linear regression analyses with the variable of interest entered as a continuous variable. Confounders considered were systolic and diastolic blood pressure, hypertension, diabetes, lipids, hypercholesterolemia, serum creatinine, body mass index, alcohol intake, current smoking status and smoking pack years.

We investigated whether the association of homocysteine with hearing was explained by markers of vascular disease and the association of B vitamins with hearing was explained by homocysteine or markers of vascular disease by subsequently adding these variables into the regression model. We included mean arterial pressure as covariates in the analyses involving distension. Because the MTHFR 677TT genotype is associated with elevated concentrations of homocysteine mainly when folate status is low, we stratified the population by the folate status (population median), and studied the relationship between genotype and hearing levels within these strata. The latter analyses were adjusted for age, sex and education level using ANCOVA. Statistical significance was defined as $p < 0.05$ (two-tailed). Statistical analyses were performed using SPSS 11.0 for Windows.

Results

Seventy-two percent of the study participants were male and the average age was 60±6 years (Table 5.1). Median homocysteine concentrations were 13.3 μmol/L (range 10.1 to 29.4 μmol/L). Nine percent, 2% and 12% of the participants had deficient levels of serum folate, erythrocyte folate and vitamin B_6 according to the American Institute of Medicine.[245] The MTHFR 677T allelic distribution did not significantly differ from the calculated expected distribution, assuming a Hardy-Weinberg equilibrium. Our study

Table 5.1 Population characteristics (*n*=729).

		Mean (standard deviation) Median (interquartile range)
Audiometry		
	PTA-high, dB[a]	34.1 (22.5 to 50.0)
	PTA-low, dB[b]	11.7 (7.5 to 17.5)
Demographics		
	Age, years	60 ± 6
	% Male	72
	% Low / Middle / High level of education	23 / 37 / 40
Markers of vascular disease		
	Carotid intima-media thickness, mm	1.02 ± 0.17
	Carotid distension, mm	0.64 ± 0.16
	% Familial history of premature vascular disease	21
	% Vascular disease	11
Clinical		
	Homocysteine, µmol/L	13.3 ± 2.9
	Serum folate, nmol/L	12 ± 4
	Erythrocyte folate, nmol/L	691 ± 260
	Vitamin B_{12}, pmol/L	287 (240 to 363)
	Vitamin B_6, nmol/L	32 (25 to 42)
	Creatinine, µmol/L	92 ± 12
	Total cholesterol, mmol/L	5.8 ± 1.1
	High-density lipoprotein cholesterol, mmol/L	1.2 ± 0.4
	Low-density lipoprotein cholesterol, mmol/L	4.0 ± 0.9
	Triglycerides, mmol/L	1.2 (0.8 to 1.6)
	% Hypercholesterolemia	35
	Systolic blood pressure, mmHg	133 ± 16
	Diastolic blood pressure, mmHg	77 ± 8
	% Hypertension	21.5
	Body mass index, kg/m^2	27 ± 4
	% Diabetes mellitus	3
Lifestyle		
	% Current smokers	20
	Folate intake, µg/d	195 (159 to 242)
	Alcohol intake, g/d	12 (4 to 24)

[a] PTA-high average pure-tone air conduction threshold at 4 kHz, 6 kHz and 8 kHz.
[b] PTA-low average pure-tone air conduction threshold at 0.5 kHz, 1 kHz and 2 kHz.

population had a higher prevalence of MTHFR 677TT homozygotes than in the general population in The Netherlands (15.7 vs. ~10%, respectively);[39] this is a likely consequence of our homocysteine and vitamin B_{12} inclusion criteria.

Table 5.2 Mean hearing thresholds in dB adjusted for age, sex and educational level per tertile of homocysteine and B vitamins concentrations (*n*=729).

		n	PTA-high[a]	PTA-low[b]
Homocysteine[c]				
	1st tertile	243	32.9	12.2
	2nd tertile	243	35.3	12.6
	3rd tertile	243	33.2	11.5
	P_{trend}		0.537	0.079
Serum folate[d]				
	1st tertile	244	32.3†	11.9
	2nd tertile	243	34.3	11.6†
	3rd tertile	242	34.9	12.8
	P_{trend}		0.023	0.090
Erythrocyte folate[e]				
	1st tertile	243	33.2	12.0
	2nd tertile	243	34.6	12.0
	3rd tertile	243	33.7	12.3
	P_{trend}		0.263	0.495
Vitamin B_{12}[f]				
	1st tertile	241	33.2*	11.7
	2nd tertile	246	32.3*	11.9
	3rd tertile	242	36.1	12.6
	P_{trend}		0.007	0.057
Vitamin B_6[g]				
	1st tertile	241	33.3	12.0
	2nd tertile	243	34.0	12.2
	3rd tertile	244	34.2	12.1
	P_{trend}		0.094	0.164

* $p<0.05$ vs. 3rd tertile.
† $p<0.10$ vs. 3rd tertile.
[a] PTA-high average pure-tone air conduction threshold at 4 kHz, 6 kHz and 8 kHz.
[b] PTA-low average pure-tone air conduction threshold at 0.5 kHz, 1 kHz and 2 kHz.
[c] Homocysteine tertiles 1: ≤13.1 μmol/L; 2: 13.2-14.7 μmol/L; 3: ≥14.8 μmol/L.
[d] Serum folate tertiles 1: ≤10.2 nmol/L; 2: 10.3-13.6 nmol/L; 3: ≥13.7 nmol/L.
[e] Erythrocyte folate tertiles 1: ≤551 nmol/L; 2: 552-754 nmol/L; 3: ≥755 nmol/L.
[f] Vitamin B_{12} tertiles 1: ≤264 pmol/L; 2: 265-347 pmol/L; 3: ≥348 pmol/L.
[g] Vitamin B_6 tertiles 1: ≤26 nmol/L; 2: 27-37 nmol/L; 3: ≥38 nmol/L.

Age, sex and educational level were the main determinants of PTA-high thresholds whereas only age and educational level were the main determinants of PTA-low hearing thresholds. These demographic factors alone could explain 25% and 12% of the variation in PTA-high and PTA-low hearing levels, respectively. Risk factors of vascular disease that have been linked to hearing loss from previous studies, such as diabetes mellitus, hypertension, smoking and hypercholesterolemia, were not independently associated with hearing thresholds. Markers of atherosclerosis and arterial stiffness were not associated with PTA-high or PTA-low. However, familial history of premature vascular disease was associated with PTA-low and PTA-high (standardized beta PTA-low 0.08, p=0.029; PTA-high 0.07, p=0.081) whereas prevalence of vascular disease was independently associated with PTA-high only (standardized beta 0.08, p=0.026).

Homocysteine, B vitamins and hearing levels

The mean age, sex and educational level adjusted hearing threshold of the low and high frequencies per tertile of homocysteine, folate, vitamin B_{12} and vitamin B_6 are given in Table 5.2. Contrary to our hypothesis, the direction of association was such that low concentrations of homocysteine and high concentrations of B vitamins were associated with elevated hearing thresholds for PTA-high and PTA-low, although this relation was statistically significant for serum folate and vitamin B_{12} only. The direct association of serum folate and vitamin B_{12} with PTA-high hearing thresholds was independent of homocysteine concentrations and other risk factors of vascular disease, including prevalent vascular disease and premature vascular disease.

MTHFR genotype and hearing levels

The MTHFR 677TT genotype was paired with higher homocysteine concentrations and lower serum folate concentrations, despite similar folate intake (Table 5.3). No other variables shown in Table 5.1 differed between the MTHFR C677T genotypes. Before adjustment for age, sex and educational level, MTHFR 677TT homozygotes had slightly lower PTA-high hearing thresholds (median [interquartile range] 30 dB [20 to 49 dB]) than subjects with the MTHFR CT and MTHFR CC genotype (CT: 36 dB, 95% CI 23 to 51 dB, TT vs. CT p=0.065; CC: 35 dB 95% CI 23 to 49 dB, TT vs. CC p=0.079). Because the phenotypic expression of the MTHFR C677T polymorphism is most pronounced when folate concentrations are low, we stratified the population based on median folate concentrations. MTHFR 677TT homozygotes with a folate status below that of the population median did not have higher hearing thresholds than CC homozygotes (Table 5.4). Because folate status is influenced by MTHFR C677T genotype, we also examined the association of MTHFR C677T genotype with hearing levels stratified by folate intake. Similarly, MTHFR 677TT homozygotes with a folate intake below that of the population did not have higher hearing thresholds than CC homozygotes.

Table 5.3 Mean homocysteine concentrations and folate status per 5,10-methylenetetrahydrofolate reductase (MTHFR) 677C→T genotype.

	Median (Interquartile range)					
MTHFR 677C→T genotype	CC *n*=280		CT *n*=331		TT *n*=114	
Homocysteine, μmol/L	13.7	(12.9 to 15.2)	13.7	(12.7 to 15.1)	14.9	(13.2 to 17.1)*
Serum folate, nmol/L	12	(10 to 15)	12	(9 to 15)†	11	(9 to 14)‡
Erythrocyte folate, nmol/L	688	(538 to 838)	611	(510 to 782)§	674	(478 to 961)
Folate intake, μg/d	198	(159 to 241)	190	(155 to 248)	200	(173 to 227)

* $p<0.001$ TT vs. CC or CT.
† $p=0.013$ CT vs. CC.
‡ $p<0.001$ CT vs. CC.
§ $p=0.004$ CT vs. CC.

It is of interest to note, that subjects in the upper half of the folate status distribution with two MTHFR 677T alleles compared with subjects with either one or no T allele tended to have on average lower hearing thresholds, although this was borderline significant. (Table 5.4). Furthermore, the association of folate status with hearing thresholds depended on MTHFR C677T genotype: high serum folate concentrations were associated with lower hearing thresholds in MTHFR 677TT homozygotes, whereas high serum folate concentrations were associated with higher hearing thresholds in MTHFR CC homozygotes (PTA-low: CC r=0.12, $p=0.033$; TT r=-0.12, $p=0.187$, adjusted for age, sex, educational level). A similar trend was seen in PTA-high, but did not reach statistical significance.

Discussion

The main findings of our study are that an elevated concentration of homocysteine, a novel risk factor for vascular disease, is not associated with hearing. Likewise, determinants of elevated concentrations of homocysteine—low concentrations of B vitamins—were not associated with elevated hearing thresholds. Conversely, high concentrations of serum folate and vitamin B_{12} were associated with poorer hearing in the high frequencies, independent of homocysteine and markers of cardiovascular disease. MTHFR 677TT homozygotes had similar hearing levels as subjects with a C allele when folate status was below the median. However, when folate status was above population median, MTHFR 677TT genotype seemed to offer protection against hearing loss.

Table 5.4 Mean hearing thresholds in dB per 5,10-methylenetetrahydrofolate reductase (MTHFR) 677C→T genotype stratified by folate status,[a] adjusted for age, sex and educational level.

	MTHFR 677C→T genotype	*n*	PTA-high[b]	PTA-low[c]
Total population				
	CC	280	34.2	12.3
	CT	331	34.0	12.2
	TT	114	32.5	11.3
	P_{trend}		0.616	0.496
Serum folate				
<50 percentile				
	CC	129	34.0	11.7
	CT	168	32.2	11.6
	TT	71	34.6	12.2
	P_{trend}		0.430	0.825
>50 percentile				
	CC	151	34.5†	12.9*
	CT	163	35.6*§	12.7*
	TT	43	29.8§	10.1§
	P_{trend}		0.069	0.055
Erythrocyte folate				
<50 percentile				
	CC	121	33.9	12.1
	CT	188	33.5	12.5
	TT	54	32.9	11.7
	P_{trend}		0.916	0.769
>50 percentile				
	CC	159	34.4	12.5
	CT	143	34.4	11.8
	TT	60	32.5	11.0
	P_{trend}		0.682	0.376
Folate intake				
<50 percentile				
	CC	132	33.2	11.7
	CT	176	32.7	11.3
	TT	55	31.5	12.1
	P_{trend}		0.792	0.726
>50 percentile				
	CC	148	35.3	12.9†
	CT	155	35.3	13.3*‡
	TT	59	33.6	10.6
	P_{trend}		0.758	0.076

* $p<0.05$ vs. TT.
† $p<0.10$ vs. TT.
‡ $p<0.05$ vs. same genotype <50 percentile.

§ $p<0.10$ vs. same genotype <50 percentile.
[a] Median cut-off. Serum folate 11.7 nmol/L, erythrocyte folate 657 nmol/L, dietary folate 195 µg/d.
[b] PTA-high average pure-tone air conduction threshold at 4 kHz, 6 kHz and 8 kHz.
[c] PTA-low average pure-tone air conduction threshold at 0.5 kHz, 1 kHz and 2 kHz.

That low concentrations of serum folate and vitamin B_{12} are independently associated with hearing acuity refutes the results of two cross-sectional populations with age-related hearing loss. With a relatively small study population (n=55), Houston and colleagues were the first to report an inverse association of erythrocyte folate and vitamin B_{12} with hearing thresholds in women, aged 60 to 71 years, in both crude and age-adjusted analyses.[102] These findings were not confirmed using data from a Danish study population (age range 67 to 88 years). In the latter study, erythrocyte folate and vitamin B_{12} concentrations were not associated with hearing thresholds in 91 patients referred to the audiological department.[103] However, in concordance with the latter study, we report a null association of homocysteine and erythrocyte folate with hearing thresholds.

In our population, high serum folate concentrations were associated with better hearing in MTHFR 677TT homozygotes, whereas high serum folate concentrations were associated with poorer hearing in CC homozygotes. Contrary to our *a priori* hypothesis, subjects with the MTHFR 677TT genotype tended to have better hearing than subjects with the 677C allele, although the differences in hearing thresholds between MTHFR C677T genotypes did not always reach statistical significance. Nevertheless, given the general pattern of our data we can speculate on the pathobiology of sensorineural hearing loss. Our data lend support to the mitochondrial damage theory of age-related hearing loss. This theory purports that damage to the mitochondrial DNA slowly builds up over time and once a critical threshold is attained, the mitochondria are rendered bioenergetically inefficient and cells undergo apoptosis.[287] A possible protective effect of the MTHFR 677TT genotype may lie in its greater relative one-carbon commitment to *de novo* synthesis of nucleotides and an increase in formyl-folate derivatives relative to methyl-folate derivatives. In theory, subjects with a greater capacity of thymidylate synthesis and 10-formyltetrahydrofolate generation may have a reduced risk of mitochondrial DNA damage in two ways. Individuals with the MTHFR 677TT genotype may have increased thymidylate synthesis that may directly reduce mitochondrial DNA mutations by ensuring a smaller pool of uracil. Secondly, MTHFR 677TT homozygotes may have greater amounts of 10-formyltetrahydrofolate, which may protect mitochondrial integrity by reducing cytochrome *c*[260] and due to its structural lability may have other antioxidant-like functions.[46]

A shift in the distribution of folate derivatives is not only influenced by polymorphisms in folate-dependent enzymes like MTHFR C677T polymorphism, but also by intracellular folate concentrations. Low folate concentrations are associated with a greater retention of one-carbon moieties for *de novo* nucleotide synthesis and greater 10-formyltetrahydrofolate concentrations.[46] Thus, in subjects with the MTHFR 677CC or 677CT genotype, lower folate concentrations may be linked to DNA fidelity and increased oxidative phosphorylation of the mitochondria, and may explain why these subjects have better hearing when folate levels are low.

It is unclear why elevated concentrations of vitamin B_{12} are associated with elevated hearing thresholds. It is clear that vitamin B_{12} deficiency is associated with neurological diseases, but little evidence exists that increasing vitamin B_{12} concentrations in non-deficient individuals improves neurological function. Perhaps at the expense of one-carbon commitment for *de novo* synthesis, high concentrations of vitamin B_{12} may push forward methylation reactions. A recent dose finding study has reported a steady decrease in homocysteine concentrations with increasing vitamin B_{12} supplementation however the effect of various vitamin B_{12} doses on folate derivatives was not examined (S Eussen. Personal communication).

Our original hypothesis was that vascular disease risk factors, elevated homocysteine and decreased folate concentrations were associated with poorer hearing, possibly independent of vascular disease. As such, we have not measured markers of mitochondrial DNA damage load or markers of mitochondrial function. These measurements, preferably from cochlear tissues, are indeed needed to support or refute our theory on the importance of MTHFR C677T polymorphism in sensorineural hearing loss.

In agreement with previous studies, prevalence of vascular disease was weakly associated with poor hearing. However, whether poor hearing precedes vascular disease or is subsequent to vascular disease has been unclear nor can be concluded from our data. Measurement of the extent and severity of atherosclerosis may lead to a more accurate risk association of hearing and vascular disease: atherosclerotic changes often precede vascular disease years before a clinical event, subsequent diet and lifestyle changes and introduction of possibly ototoxic drug regimens. However, in our population neither carotid intima-media thickness nor distension was related to hearing thresholds. Our findings do not support a strong role for vascular disease in the etiology of age-related hearing loss.

This study is a cross-sectional study. Therefore we cannot presume that an increase in folate concentrations might be beneficial for MTHFR 677TT homozygotes or detrimental for CC homozygotes. Our findings need to be confirmed in other populations that do not screen participants on characteristics influenced by MTHFR 677TT genotype, like homocysteine concentrations. Nevertheless, when we stratified our data based on folate intake, which we expect is not directly influenced by MTHFR C677T genotype, similar, but less pronounced, associations of folate with hearing levels were found.

The actual clinical significance associated with a maximal difference of 5 dB between MTHFR 677TT subjects with low and high serum folate status is quite substantial. Recent evidence from Epidemiology of Hearing Loss Study in Beaver Dam, Wisconsin has shown that over a period of five years, more than half of the subjects with impaired hearing (PTA >25 dB for 0.5, 1, 2 and 4 kHz) experienced ≥5 dB increase in hearing thresholds.[312] Larger epidemiological studies are required to determine how environmental and genetic factors that influence one-carbon metabolism affect hearing. We are currently conducting a trial examining the effect of three-year supplementation with 0.8 mg/d folic acid on markers of vascular disease, cognitive function and hearing thresholds; we expect to report our findings in 2005.[48]

Chapter 6

One-year folic acid supplementation does not affect inflammation markers in middle-aged and elderly: a randomized controlled trial

Jane Durga, L.J.H. van Tits, Evert G. Schouten, Frans J. Kok, Petra Verhoef

Division of Human Nutrition, Wageningen University, Wageningen, The Netherlands
Wageningen Centre for Food Sciences, Wageningen, The Netherlands
Department of General Internal Medicine, University Medical Center Nijmegen, Nijmegen, The Netherlands

Submitted

Abstract

Background Elevated concentrations of homocysteine and low concentrations of folate may lead to a proinflammatory state that could explain their relation with cardiovascular disease risk.

Aim We investigated the effect of homocysteine-lowering by folic acid supplementation (0.8 mg/d) on markers of inflammation.

Methods In a double blind randomized placebo-controlled trial among 530 men and post-menopausal women, with homocysteine concentrations ≥13 µmol/L at screening, we investigated the effect of folic acid supplementation (0.8 mg/d) versus placebo for one year on C-reactive protein, soluble intercellular adhesion molecule-1, oxidized low-density lipoprotein (LDL) and autoantibodies against oxidized LDL.

Results After one year of supplementation, concentrations of serum folate increased by 430% and homocysteine decreased by 25% in the folic acid group compared with the placebo group. However, no changes in plasma concentrations of the inflammation markers were observed.

Conclusion Although homocysteine is associated with vascular disease risk in the general population, marked lowering of slightly elevated homocysteine concentrations by one-year folic acid supplementation does not influence inflammatory responses involving C-reactive protein, soluble intercellular adhesion molecule-1, oxidized LDL and autoantibodies against oxidized LDL.

Introduction

Homocysteine is an independent risk factor for cardiovascular disease. Inflammation has been implicated in atherosclerosis and cardiovascular disease[313,314] and may partly explain the association of homocysteine with cardiovascular disease. Homocysteine has been associated with a proinflammatory response in *in vitro*, in animal models and in humans. In rats elevated concentrations of homocysteine have been associated with increased carotid artery permeability, which may affect low-density lipoprotein (LDL) intravasation and accumulation in the arterial wall.[246] Trapped LDL interacts with reactive oxygen species to form minimally oxidized LDL, which stimulates the expression of adhesion molecules, chemotactic proteins and growth factors. Indeed, elevated concentrations of homocysteine have been associated with increased concentrations of monocyte chemotactic protein-1 and increased expression of adhesion molecules in rats[315-317] and in humans.[318,319] In addition, homocysteine-lowering via folic acid supplementation ameliorated these effects.[315-319] Upon further oxidation, the highly oxidized LDL is taken up by macrophages and vascular smooth muscle cells to form foam cells, which make up the fatty deposits of initial lesions. Dead foam cells form the necrotic core of more advanced plaque, which upon rupture releases oxidized LDL, cytokines, chemokines and clotting factors into the blood stream. In line with this, hyperhomocysteinemia has been associated with advanced atherosclerosis[215,219,233] and in humans, treatment with B vitamins appears to hinder plaque progression.[62,63]

In a randomized placebo-controlled trial we investigated whether homocysteine-reduction through daily folic acid supplementation (0.8 mg) leads to decreased concentrations of markers of the inflammatory response, i.e. C-reactive protein, soluble intercellular adhesion molecule-1, oxidized LDL and autoantibodies against oxidized LDL.

Methods

Subjects

Data come from men and post-menopausal women aged 50 to 70 years from the Gelderland region in The Netherlands participating in the Folic Acid and Carotid Intima-media Thickness (FACIT) study, a trial investigating whether folic acid supplementation can halt the progression of atherosclerosis. Data was collected from the last 530 of the 819 subjects of the FACIT study between February 2000 and December 2002. Major exclusion criteria were homocysteine <13 µmol/L, vitamin B_{12} <200 pmol/L, renal or thyroid diseases, use of B vitamin supplements or medications that influence folate metabolism or atherosclerotic progression (e.g. lipid-lowering and hormone replacement therapies) and <80% self-reported compliance during a six-week run-in period. The Medical Ethics Committee of Wageningen University approved the study and subjects gave written informed consent.

Design

The sequence of entry into the study was randomly allocated to either treatment using permuted blocks with block sizes of four and six (computer generated randomization list was kindly provided by Dr. Huub P.J. Willems (Department of Haematology, Leyenburg Hospital, The Hague, The Netherlands). The sequence number served also as the participant's allocation code, thus each participant had a unique code so as to decrease the chance of unmasking by the investigator. After the measurement sessions, subjects were allocated to treatment with folic acid or placebo in capsule-form. The capsules were specially produced by Swiss Caps Benelux (Roosendaal, The Netherlands). Capsules were individually packaged in foil pill strips containing 28 pills per strip, the days of the week were printed on the back of the strips to aid compliance and registration. The capsules were indistinguishable in appearance (yellow coating and content) and taste. Members of the same household received the same intervention to avoid contamination or comparisons between pills. Blinding for the participants appeared successful: at the completion of the three-year trial in a sample of 260 participants, 60% did not know which treatment they had had, 10% suspected folic acid treatment and 30% suspected placebo treatment. These suspicions were equally distributed across the folic acid and placebo groups. Research assistants allocating treatment, distributing treatment and collecting blood were blinded to group assignment. During the trial, compliance (defined as >80% of capsules taken) was judged by pill-return counts and a calendar that registered missed pills, both returned every twelve weeks. Fasting venous blood was collected in K3 EDTA (1 mg/mL) vacutainer tubes for determination of inflammation markers for this sub-trial in the last 530 subjects at the time of randomization and after one year (± six weeks). Plasma was isolated immediately by centrifugation and, after addition of saccharose (final concentration 0.6%) to prevent denaturation of lipoproteins during freezing, was stored in aliquots at -80°C until analyses.

Blood measurements

We measured plasma C-reactive protein by a commercially available ELISA (Dako, Glastrup, Denmark) according to the instructions of the manufacturer. The intra-assay CV was 6.0% and inter-assay CV was 9.7%. Plasma soluble intercellular adhesion molecule-1 was measured with a sandwich ELISA described elsewhere.[320] Monoclonal antibody HM2 was used as the capture antibody and biotin-labeled monoclonal antibody HM1 as the detection antibody. The lower detection limit of the assay was 400 pg/mL. The intra-assay CV was 2.7% and inter-assay CV was 9.1%. Plasma oxidized LDL was measured with a sandwich ELISA, using the monoclonal antibody 4E6 as the capture antibody and anti-human apoB-100 polyclonal antibody as the detection antibody. Monoclonal antibody 4E6 attaches to a conformational epitope in the apoB-100 moiety of LDL that is generated as a consequence of aldehyde substitution of lysine residues of apoB-100[321] and is considered specific for oxidatively modified LDL. Autoantibodies against oxidized LDL were measured as described previously.[322]

Plasma total homocysteine concentrations were determined with HPLC and fluorimetric detection.[242] Serum folate and vitamin B_{12} were measured using a chemiluminescent immunoassay (Immulite® 2000, Diagnostic Products Corporation). Erythrocyte folate was determined in duplicate and the average was taken to reduce measurement error. Serum creatinine and lipids were determined using Hitachi® 747 analyzer (Roche). We defined hypercholesterolemia as total cholesterol >6.5 mmol/L, high-density lipoprotein cholesterol cholesterol <0.9 mmol/L or use of lipid-lowering medication. The 5,10-methylenetetrahydrofolate reductase (MTHFR) 677C→T polymorphism was determined by polymerase chain reaction of DNA and restriction enzyme digestion with *Hin*Fl.

Other measurements

A self-reported medical history, including current drug use and family history of premature vascular disease (onset <60 years in first degree family), and smoking were attained by questionnaire and reviewed by a research assistant. A participant was considered to have prevalent vascular disease if he had been diagnosed with angina pectoris, myocardial infarction, arrhythmia, stroke, or peripheral arterial disease or if he had undergone certain procedures (balloon angioplasty, coronary bypass surgery or aortic aneurysm surgery). Height and weight were measured and body mass index (kg/m^2) was calculated. Blood pressure was measured using an automated meter (Dinamap® Compact Pro 100, General Electric) in supine position, while the participant underwent the ultrasound examination. The average of eight measurements was taken. We defined hypertension as systolic blood pressure ≥160 mmHg, diastolic blood pressure ≥95 mmHg or use of antihypertensive medication. A food frequency questionnaire estimated folate intake and alcohol intake in the past three months.

Statistical analysis

Statistical analysis was performed using SPSS 11.0 for Windows. For each participant, we averaged the homocysteine concentrations measured at screening and at baseline and used this average in the analyses. Descriptive data are shown as mean ± standard deviation or median (interquartile range) depending on the distribution of the data. Skewed data were (natural log) transformed. Pearson correlations were used to examine the relation between folate and homocysteine concentrations on the one hand with markers of inflammation on the other hand in the total population at baseline. Differences in concentrations of the markers of inflammation after one-year supplementation between treatment groups were tested by *t* test. We followed the intention-to-treat principle and used baseline concentrations for post-treatment values of the inflammation markers when a subject prematurely discontinued the study. Analysis of variance was used to investigate whether the MTHFR C677T polymorphism influenced treatment effect. Statistical significance was defined as $p < 0.05$ (two-tailed). Data analysis was conducted without knowledge of the treatment code, and to retain blinding, data were assigned fake participant numbers. Researchers were denied access to the original database of study values and participant numbers.

Results

Of the 530 subjects enrolled, five subjects and four subjects allocated to the folic acid and placebo treatment, respectively, did not return for the measurements at one year. All subjects, except two, reported consumption of more than 90% of the capsules, as judged from self-reported compliance or from capsule strip return. The lowest compliance reported over a three-month period was 52%. Randomization was successful as concentrations of homocysteine, folate and inflammation markers and their determinants were similarly distributed across the folic acid (n=264) and the placebo (n=266) groups (Table 6.1). The MTHFR 677T allelic distribution did not significantly differ from the calculated expected distribution, assuming a Hardy-Weinberg equilibrium (Table 6.1).

At baseline, homocysteine and erythrocyte folate were weakly correlated with soluble intercellular adhesion molecule-1 (r=0.10, p=0.025; r=-0.10, p=0.026, respectively) and erythrocyte folate was also weakly correlated with oxidized LDL (r=-0.10, p=0.035) in crude analyses. As shown in Table 6.2, one-year supplementation with 0.8 mg/d folic acid was associated with a 430% increase in serum folate and a 25% decrease in homocysteine concentrations. However, folic acid treatment did not affect

Table 6.1 Mean (standard deviation) or median (interquartile range) values of characteristics of the folic acid and placebo group at the start of the study.[a]

	Folic acid (*n*=264)	Placebo (*n*=266)
Age, years	60 ± 5	60 ± 6
Sex, % Male	70.1	73.7
Homocysteine, µmol/L	13.9 (12.9 to 15.1)	13.9 (12.7 to 15.5)
Serum folate, nmol/L	11 (9 to 14)	11 (9 to 15)
Erythrocyte folate, nmol/L	620 (486 to 832)	677 (540 to 833)
Folate intake, µg/d	186 (156 to 230)	202 (161 to 250)
Vitamin B_{12}, pmol/L	289 (248 to 367)	288 (246 to 363)
Vitamin B_6, pmol/L	32 (25 to 41)	31 (24 to 40)
MTHFR 677C→T genotype, % CC / CT / TT	35.0 / 47.5 / 17.5	45.1 / 41.3 / 13.6
C-reactive protein, ng/L	1.5 (0.7 to 3.1)	1.1 (0.6 to 2.4)
sICAM-1, µg/L	139 (118 to 160)	139 (114 to 165)
Oxidized LDL, U/L	52 (39 to 70)	52 (40 to 68)
Oxidized LDL / LDL ratio, U/mmol	13 (10 to 18)	13 (10 to 18)
IgG against oxidized LDL, OD_{450}	0.15 (0.09 to 0.22)	0.14 (0.08 to 0.24)
IgM against oxidized LDL, OD_{450}	0.13 (0.07 to 0.23)	0.14 (0.08 to 0.24)
Total cholesterol, mmol/L	5.9 ± 1.1	5.9 ± 1.2
High-density lipoprotein cholesterol, mmol/L	1.2 ± 0.3	1.3 ± 0.4
Low-density lipoprotein cholesterol, mmol/L	4.1 ± 1.0	4.1 ± 1.1
Hypercholesterolemia, %	42.4	36.8
Systolic blood pressure, mmHg	133 ± 16	133 ± 17
Hypertension, %	22	20
Creatinine, µmol/L	91 ± 12	93 ± 12
Alcohol intake, g/d	13 (4 to 24)	13 (5 to 23)
Body mass index, kg/m^2	27 ± 3	27 ± 4
Current smoking, %	22.0	18.4
Diabetes mellitus, %	2.3	4.1
Prevalent vascular disease, %	15.5	9.8

[a] Abbreviations. MTHFR 5,10-methylenetetrahydrofolate reductase 677C→T polymorphism; sICAM-1 soluble intercellular adhesion molecule-1; LDL low-density lipoprotein; OD_{450} optical density at 450 nm.

concentrations of the inflammation markers. Nor did lipid parameters change due to treatment (data not shown).

At baseline, homocysteine concentrations were 8% higher and serum folate concentrations were 18% lower in MTHFR 677TT homozygotes compared with subjects with the CC genotype. Concentrations of inflammation markers did not differ between the genotypes (data not shown). Furthermore, MTHFR 677C→T genotype did not appear to modify the effect of folic acid supplementation on markers of inflammation after one year (data not shown).

Discussion

In this one-year randomized placebo-controlled trial, marked reduction of slightly elevated homocysteine concentrations through daily folic acid supplementation did not affect plasma concentrations of oxidized LDL, autoantibodies against oxidized LDL, soluble intercellular adhesion molecule-1 or C-reactive protein in an elderly population with a median dietary folate intake below that of the Dutch RDA (300 μg/d). Although homocysteine is associated with vascular disease risk in the general population, it is unlikely that homocysteine or folic acid act by influencing these markers of inflammation.

This randomized controlled trial is the largest trial to date, and, in line with two previous studies, did not detect a decrease in concentrations of C-reactive protein following homocysteine-lowering.[109,110] Furthermore, to our knowledge, our study is the first to report an absence of effect of folic acid supplementation on soluble intercellular adhesion molecule-1. Other adhesion molecules like vascular cell adhesion molecule-1 and E-selectin did not respond to two-year supplementation with a combination of folic acid and pyridoxine.[110] Upon homocysteine elevation, concentrations of vascular cellular adhesion molecule-1,[318] but not P-selectin,[323] concomitantly increased hours after methionine loading. In the former study, whether this increase was significant relative to control group is unclear.

There is considerable evidence that C-reactive protein, soluble intercellular adhesion molecule-1 and oxidized LDL are involved in atherosclerosis[314,324] and predict risk of cardiovascular disease,[325,326] although, longitudinal studies on the association of oxidized LDL with cardiovascular disease risk are more scarce.[327] Formation of oxidized LDL *in vivo* leads to the generation of autoantibodies against various forms of oxidized LDL. Findings from experimental and epidemiological research on the relation of autoantibodies against oxidized LDL with atherosclerosis or cardiovascular disease are inconsistent. Plasma levels of autoantibodies against oxidized LDL correlate with amount of oxidized LDL in lesions, have been associated with risk of cardiovascular disease,[328,329] although not consistently[330] and localize to atherosclerotic lesions *in vivo.*[324] The mechanism via which autoantibodies against oxidized LDL influence atherosclerosis is not clear but may involve clearance of atherogenic oxidatively modified LDL. IgG autoantibodies against oxidized LDL were shown to induce macrophage Fcγ receptor-mediated phagocytosis of oxidized LDL.[331] On the other hand, autoantibodies against oxidized LDL may block uptake of oxidized LDL by macrophages.[332,333] Moreover, oxi-

Table 6.2 Median (interquartile range) concentrations of serum folate, plasma homocysteine and inflammation markers after one-year treatment with folic acid or placebo.[a]

	Folic acid	Placebo	p value[b]
Serum folate, nmol/L	60 (45 to 85)	12 (10 to 15)	<0.001
Homocysteine, µmol/L	9.1 (8.1 to 10.5)	12.6 (10.9 to 14.8)	<0.001
C-reactive protein, mg/L	1.4 (0.9 to 3.1)	1.2 (0.6 to 3.1)	0.883
sICAM-1, µg/L	139 (119 to 161)	139 (118 to 170)	0.688
Oxidized LDL, U/L	53 (39 to 71)	55 (41 to 70)	0.918
Oxidized LDL /LDL ratio, U/mmol	14 (10 to 19)	14 (10 to 19)	0.898
IgG against oxidized LDL, OD_{450}	0.12 (0.08 to 0.21)	0.13 (0.07 to 0.26)	0.393
IgM against oxidized LDL, OD_{450}	0.13 (0.07 to 0.23)	0.13 (0.08 to 0.23)	0.116

[a] Abbreviations. sICAM-1 soluble intercellular adhesion molecule-1; LDL low-density lipoprotein; OD_{450} optical density at 450 nm.
[b] We used the *t* test to test whether the (natural log) transformed mean concentration after 1 year differed between the groups, based on intention-to-treat principles.

datively modified LDL has been found to bind to innate pattern recognition receptors such as CD14 and C-reactive protein and activate toll-like receptor 4, which could enhance macrophage function and atherogenesis.[334]

In our population, erythrocyte folate but not homocysteine was weakly inversely related to oxidized LDL, however, folic acid supplementation did not affect concentrations of oxidized LDL or autoantibodies against oxidized LDL. These findings concur with trials in the general population or in patients with coronary disease, which found no effect of B vitamin supplementation on *in vitro* LDL oxidizability or plasma malondialdehyde, a final product of lipid peroxidation.[105-107] Likewise, folic acid supplementation in combination with vitamin B_{12} did not decrease urinary levels of 8-epi-prostagladin $F_{2\alpha}$, an indicator of oxidative stress, in subjects with cognitive impairment.[100] In renal patients, however, oxidative stress appears responsive to high doses of folic acid or folinic acid therapy. In these patients, a 40-50% decrease in homocysteine concentrations was associated with a 30-40% reduction in serum and erythrocyte malondialdehyde concentrations and a 13% reduction in autoantibodies against oxidized LDL.[335-337] These trials did not employ a placebo-controlled arm and hence should be interpreted with caution. In our study a comparable decrease in homocysteine concentrations was found (25% decrease), and the decrease in subjects with the MTHFR 677TT genotype was even greater (40% decrease). Nevertheless, concentrations of the inflammation markers did not respond to folic acid in subjects with the MTHFR 677TT genotype, similar to earlier findings,[106] or in subjects in the upper half of the homocysteine distribution (data not shown). Although the relative reduction was similar, the renal patients post-intervention concentrations of homocysteine were much higher compared with our own study (~20 vs. 9 µmol/L, respectively). One study in the general population has shown a decrease in C-reactive protein concentrations after multi-vitamin supplementation, which included 0.8 mg folic acid, however the effect was greater in subjects with initial C-reactive protein concentrations ≥1 mg/L.[338] However, even when we confined our analyses to those subjects in the upper half of the distribution of the inflammation markers or in the lower half of the folate distribution our results did not change (data not shown).

Were we too late in intervening, was the duration not long enough or is folic acid an inappropriate intervention? We have shown that one-year folic acid supplementation in the elderly (mean age 65 years) did not lead to an improvement in markers of inflammation despite a marked decrease in homocysteine. The trials in renal patients that observed reductions in autoantibodies against oxidized LDL and malondialdehyde were shorter than our trial (three to six months).[335-337] Furthermore, a two-year trial in subjects younger than our population did not detect differences in C-reactive protein and adhesion molecules (mean age 47 years). Whether a dietary folate approach or supplemental folic acid may determine the success of homocysteine-lowering on inflammatory markers is unclear. Adhering to a folate-rich diet for sixteen weeks, compared with folic acid or control diet, did not affect malondialdehyde concentrations.[106] However, in patients with coronary artery disease, a whole grain diet compared with the white-rice control was associated with a decrease in homocysteine and malondialdehyde concentrations after sixteen weeks.[339]

The possible pathogenic mechanism of elevated concentrations of homocysteine in cardiovascular disease remains unclear. Elevated concentrations of homocysteine and decreased concentrations of folate may have proinflammatory properties in the elderly;[319] however, their amelioration through folic acid supplementation is unlikely to influence C-reactive protein, soluble intercellular adhesion molecule-1 and oxidized LDL, directly. We must await the large secondary prevention trials to evaluate whether B vitamin supplementation indeed leads to less cardiovascular disease.

Chapter 7

Discussion

The main objectives of this thesis were to describe the relationship between folate and homocysteine, on the one hand, with markers of cardiovascular disease risk, cognitive performance and hearing thresholds, on the other hand, using data from the FACIT study participants at baseline. Furthermore, we studied the effect of supplementation with folic acid on reduction in plasma concentrations of inflammation markers after one-year in the FACIT study participants. In this chapter we discuss how our findings on the association of folate and homocysteine with risk of cardiovascular disease, cognitive performance and hearing impairment add to the understanding of the etiology of cardiovascular disease, age-related cognitive decline and age-related hearing loss, respectively, in the middle-aged and elderly. Drawing on our findings, we suggest promising research areas that will further our understanding of these age-related conditions and discuss implications for public health policy.

Cardiovascular disease risk

Low concentrations of folate were weakly associated with increased risk of cardiovascular disease as measured by carotid artery intima-media thickness, a valid surrogate marker of cardiovascular disease risk and a structural marker of atherosclerosis (Chapter 3).[57] The association was independent of conventional risk factors for vascular disease and homocysteine concentrations (Chapter 3). Similar to our own results, large observational studies have shown an inverse association between folate status and clinically relevant endpoints such as cardiovascular morbidity and mortality.[36] However, we were the first research group to detect an inverse association between folate and carotid intima-media thickness, perhaps because other study populations had an adequate folate status (Chapter 2). Ten percent of our study population was deficient in folate, a likely consequence of our inclusion criterion for slightly elevated concentrations of homocysteine. Evidence from two randomized controlled trials—one in renal transplant recipients and the other in vascular disease patients—shows that folic acid supplementation, in combination with other B vitamins, leads to regression of the carotid intima-media thickness.[54,55]

Hyperhomocysteinemia, on the other hand, was not associated with vascular disease risk, as measured by carotid intima-media thickness (Chapter 3). Our results are in line with the vast majority of studies, which have found no association of elevated concentrations of homocysteine with carotid intima-media thickness (Chapter 2). This suggests that previous observational studies, which examined the association of homocysteine and clinical end points of vascular disease may be explained by reverse causality, as carotid intima-media thickening occurs years before complications associated with advanced atherosclerosis become clinically evident. Alternatively, the pathogenic mechanisms associated with hyperhomocysteinemia may not affect atherosclerosis, but other processes often associated with atherosclerosis such as thrombosis.

In 1962, the clinical significance of homocysteine was discovered when two research groups simultaneously reported venous thrombosis and other vascular abnormalities in patients with severely elevated concentrations of homocysteine.[340,341] These patients were later discovered to have inborn errors in the metabolism of homocysteine.[342] In these patients, treatment with B vitamins has reduced the risk of thromboembolic disease.[124] However, in patients with hyperhomocysteinemia, treatment with B vitamins did not decrease the recurrence of deep venous thrombosis or lung embolism compared with patients taking the placebo (relative risk 0.8, 95% CI 0.6 to 1.3; M den Heijer. Personal communication). High concentrations of homocysteine have been also associated with arterial thrombosis, both in the general population and in vascular disease patients.[50] Arterial thrombosis, however, often occurs in subjects with advanced atherosclerosis; thus, it is impossible to disentangle the relative contribution of advanced atherosclerosis from arterial thrombosis when using clinical endpoints such as myocardial infarction or transient ischemic attack. High concentrations of homocysteine have been associated with an imbalance in hemostasis markers, favoring thrombogenesis.[343] However, experimental studies with vascular disease patients or in the general population have led to inconsistent results on the effect of B vitamins on markers of hemostasis (see references therein).[109] In the FACIT trial, one-year supplementation with folic acid did not influence markers of hemostasis involved in either the pro-coagulation or fibrinolytic pathways.[109]

The lack of association between homocysteine and vascular disease risk may be because high homocysteine concentrations affect the arterial wall in other ways than carotid intima-media thickening. The effects of hyperhomocysteinemia on the thickening of the intima and media walls are inconsistent in animal models and have been relatively unexplored in humans.[219,220,233,248] The only morphological distinction in the femoral arteries between peripheral arterial disease patients with or without hyperhomocysteinemia was a decreased medial smooth muscle cell / extracellular matrix ratio, which may lead to an increase in arterial stiffness.[221] These changes cannot be detected by carotid intima-media thickness. However, we show that neither folate nor homocysteine are associated with carotid distension, a marker of arterial stiffness

(Chapter 3). This is in agreement with other observational studies conducted in the general population, showing no association between homocysteine and markers of arterial stiffness.[85,87]

Recent evidence suggests that high concentrations of homocysteine lead to greater plaque progression and treatment with B vitamins may slow down the rate of progression in patients with unexplained advanced atherosclerosis.[62] Although carotid intima-media thickness and plaque prevalence are correlated, measurement of plaque size may better capture a relation, if any, with homocysteine than arterial wall thickening. Therefore, we have included plaque measurements in the final year of the FACIT trial. The results shall be presented in 2005. The future holds more advanced non-invasive techniques for imaging of atherosclerosis, such as the visualization of plaque composition with magnetic resonance imaging using contrast agents that depict macrophage activity. These techniques may enable us better study the possible atherogenic actions associated with low concentrations of folate or high concentrations of homocysteine.

Although the precise mechanism remains unclear, folate may be protective against vascular disease because of its possible antioxidant capacities, independent of homocysteine-lowering.[208] Oxidative stress leads to endothelial dysfunction and an inflammation response, forming the initial stages of atherogenesis. Folate can reduce reactive oxygen species generation by endothelial nitric oxide synthase,[105,308] ameliorate homocysteine-mediated oxidation of low-density lipoprotein (LDL)[344] and endothelial dysfunction.[108] Support for an antioxidant mechanism comes from similar studies which show that, like folate, other antioxidants such as vitamin C can limit homocysteine-mediated markers of LDL oxidation[345] and improve homocysteine-mediated endothelial dysfunction.[346] Subsequent hyperhomocysteinemia due to low concentrations of folate may also enhance oxidation, although its oxidative effects on e.g. LDL are uncertain. Whereas some studies find that homocysteine is a pro-oxidant to LDL, other studies show that it protects LDL from oxidation (and references therein).[347] Nevertheless, folic acid supplementation and subsequent homocysteine-lowering did not affect concentrations of plasma oxidized LDL or autoantibodies against oxidized LDL (Chapter 6), in agreement with other randomized controlled trials which investigated the effect of folic acid on markers of LDL oxidation.[105-107] Nor does folic acid supplementation and subsequent homocysteine-lowering affect concentrations of plasma inflammation markers such as C-reactive protein and soluble intercellular adhesion molecule-1 (Chapter 6). More promising results on markers of oxidation and inflammation have come from trials that employ dietary interventions or multivitamin supplements rather than just folic acid or the B vitamins.[107,338,339,348] This suggests that other factors that commonly vary with folate intake may explain the antioxidant or anti-inflammatory role of folate. Finally, low concentrations of folate and high concentrations of homocysteine may affect cardiovascular risk through other oxidative or inflammatory mechanisms, like upregulation of NF-κB[215,315]—a transcriptional factor central to the inflammatory response—and upregulation of macrophage-bound lectin-like oxidized LDL receptor.[319] The anti-inflammatory properties of agents that decrease homocysteine concentrations presumably without affecting folate concentrations will help disentangle whether a beneficial effect of homocysteine-lowering is independent of folate.

Neurodegenerative disorders

Cognitive performance

Low concentrations of folate were associated with poor cognitive performance, independent of vascular disease and its risk factors, including homocysteine (Chapter 4). High concentrations of homocysteine were associated with poor cognitive performance as well. Although low folate and high homocysteine concentrations were associated with poor cognitive performance, the 5,10-methylenetetrahydrofolate reductase (MTHFR) 677TT genotype was associated with better cognitive function. This finding was unexpected, as subjects with the MTHFR 677TT genotype tended to have higher homocysteine concentrations than subjects with a MTHFR 677C allele.

There is a vast, but inconsistent literature on the relation between folate and cognitive outcome measures. The late Dr. Herbert was one of the first researchers to describe the link between folate and cognition, be it in a '*n*=1' study. He subjected himself to a folate-deficient diet for three months, after which he reported feelings of paranoia, irritability and forgetfulness. These feelings resided once folates were replenished in his diet.[251] Likewise, supplementation with folate has been associated with improved cognitive performance and general mental function in patients with deficient levels of B vitamins and in patients with inborn errors of the one-carbon metabolism.[252-259] Even low, but not deficient, levels of folate have been associated with cognitive performance. In 1983, Goodwin and colleagues were the first to demonstrate an association of folate status with cognitive performance in the general population.[349] Since then, many cross-sectional and longitudinal studies have reported on the relation between folate and cognitive performance in the general population.[92,93] The low suitability of tests, often small sample sizes and type of analyses (i.e. linear vs. extreme percentile analyses) may explain the often disparate results of the studies. Whether correction of low levels of folate or high levels of homocysteine via folic acid supplementation will improve cognitive performance is inconclusive. Many trials employed small study populations, lacked a control group or placebo treatment, allocated multiple interventions such that the effect of folic acid supplementation could not be delineated or used inappropriate tests.[47,95-99] Many of the large secondary prevention studies which examine the effect of homocysteine-lowering on cardiovascular disease endpoints will include measures of cognitive function, albeit obtuse measures like the Mini-Mental State Examination,[275] a test commonly used for dementia screening (R Clarke. Personal communication).

Hearing

Folate, not homocysteine, was directly associated with hearing impairment, however, this association was confined to subjects with the MTHFR 677C allele (Chapter 5). These results are unexpected and are not in line with the two previous studies, which examined the association of folate or homocysteine with hearing levels in individuals with age-related hearing loss. The first study detected an inverse association in a small study sample of American women: high concentrations of folate were correlated with hearing acuity.[102] The second study, a Danish study, did not detect an association between folate or homocysteine and hearing levels in subjects referred to an audiology department.[103] Furthermore, animal studies have shown that deficiencies in vitamins B_{12} and B_6 and *para*-aminobenzoic acid have been associated with demyelinization of the auditory neurological tissue and other cochlear malformations.[309] No studies have been conducted that examine the effect of folate-deficient diets on cochlear morphology or hearing in animal models.

Mechanisms of folate action for neurodegeneration

Most research on the possible involvement of folate in the etiology of neurodegeneration has concentrated on the homocysteine-raising effect of folate deficiency. Low concentrations of folate and high concentrations of homocysteine may promote neurodegenerative changes in several ways by affecting the neuron directly: oxidative stress,[350,351] enhancement of β-amyloid peptide-dependent neurotoxicity,[351-353] impairment of DNA repair mechanisms,[352] including down regulation of DNA repair gene expression,[354] loss of mitochondrial membrane potential[355] and neuronal apoptosis.[356] Homocysteine may have direct toxic effects on neurons, e.g. though overexcitation of N-methyl-D-aspartate receptors.[305] Mattson and Shea provide an overview of possible pathogenic mechanisms of folate deprivation and subsequent extracellular accumulation of homocysteine for neurodegenerative disorders.[357] Aberrations to the vessels that supply the brain and cochlea may disrupt the transfer of essential nutrients and removal of toxic metabolites. Folate deficiency or subsequent hyperhomocysteinemia have been associated with degeneration of the endothelium and brain-blood barrier,[358] cerebral microangiography,[359] anti-angiogenic changes[360,361] and cerebrovascular disease.[32] Unfortunately, no research has focused on the possible adverse effects of low concentrations of folate and increased concentrations of homocysteine on cochlear cells or the stria vascularis. The question remains whether hyperhomocysteinemia *per se* or other factors involved in folate metabolism are responsible for the putative effects associated with folate deficiency. In support of the latter, observations in patients with severe MTHFR deficiency compared with patients with severe cystathionine β-synthase deficiency have more pronounced neurological pathologies, despite lower concentrations of homocysteine.[362]

Apart from hyperhomocysteinemia, changes in methylation status may be interrelated to aberrations in folate metabolism. The hypomethylation theory of neurocognitive decline, originally brought forth by Osmond and Smythies,[280] is based on the premise that low levels of folate or high levels of homocysteine result in inhibition of *S*-adenosylmethionine biosynthesis, the major methyl donor in our body, or inhibition of methyltransferase reactions (see Figure 1.1). Methylation reactions are necessary for a variety of physiological reactions in our central nervous system e.g. neurotransmitter biosynthesis. Support for the hypomethylation theory comes from studies that show depressed *S*-adenosylmethionine concentrations in patients with neurological and psychiatric disorders, the amelioration of depressive symptoms upon *S*-adenosylmethionine therapy, the enhancement of anti-depressive therapy when co-supplemented with folic acid (see Calvaresi and Bryan for review).[92] Therapies with betaine, a methyl donor which has been shown to decrease homocysteine concentrations and increase *S*-adenosylmethionine concentrations in cerebrospinal fluid,[282,363] have been shown to alleviate neurological symptoms in patients with low or undetectable levels of MTHFR activity[282] and improve cognitive performance.[283] Application of methionine to the round window of the inner ear during cancer therapy with ototoxic anti-folate agents is able to protect the ear from sensorineural hearing loss.[364,365] Whether the effect of methionine, a precursor to *S*-adenosylmethionine, is due to an increase in methylation capacity is uncertain. Other cellular changes take place when *S*-adenosylmethionine concentrations increase. For example, a shift in the distribution of folate derivatives is expected to take place, as *S*-adenosylmethionine is an allosteric inhibitor of MTHFR. The effects of MTHFR inhibition may include an accumulation of 5,10-methylenetetrahydrofolate, a molecule central to allocation of one-carbon metabolism between the cytosol and the mitochondria,[366] increase in one-carbon moieties for *de novo* nucleotide synthesis and an increase in formyl folate derivatives (see Figure 1.1). The inhibition of MTHFR may explain why methionine treatment is effective in alleviating the biochemical symptoms in patients with B_{12} deficiency thought to be due to the 'methyl trap.'[367]

This shift in folate derivatives distribution due to *S*-adenosylmethionine may be similar to that seen in subjects with the MTHFR 677TT genotype. Subjects with the MTHFR 677TT have a decreased MTHFR activity compared with the wild type enzyme as suggested by *in vitro* studies.[202] MTHFR 677TT homozygotes compared with CC homozygotes are thought to have a higher formyl : methyl tetrahydrofolate derivative ratio,[207] and presumed, therefore, to have a lower methylation capacity as indicated by elevated concentrations of homocysteine. Conversely, higher cytosolic 10-formyltetrahydrofolate concentrations may salvage mitochondrial bioenergetic efficiency[260] and in cancer tissues has been associated with decreased cytotoxicity[270] and apoptosis.[271]

Perhaps the consequences associated with a reduced activity of the MTHFR in subjects with the 677TT genotype may help explain our unexpected findings regarding the association of MTHFR 677TT genotype with neurodegenerative conditions. We found that subjects with the MTHFR 677TT genotype performed better on cognitive tests and had better hearing compared with subjects with the MTHFR 677C allele. This may be a chance finding, a result of our screening criteria or may reflect a real association and, therefore, may lead to insight into the etiology of neurodegenerative processes. Assuming that reduced activity of MTHFR is associated with increased DNA fidelity and mitochondrial bioenergetic efficiency due to an increase in one-carbon moieties for *de novo* nucleotide synthesis and an increase in 10-formyltetrahydrofolate synthesis, our findings support the mitochondrial DNA damage theory of age-related hearing loss[287] and the mitochondrial decay theory of age-related cognitive decline.[368] Few studies have reported on the nature of the association of MTHFR C677T polymorphism with cognitive function. These studies were not able to detect an association between MTHFR C677T polymorphism with high intelligence in children[272,273] or in older adults.[273] No studies have examined the association between MTHFR genotype and hearing levels.

How can we rectify our own unexpected findings that low folate status was associated with better hearing in subjects with the MTHFR 677C allele? Researchers have speculated that the activity of the enzymes involved in folate metabolism depend in part on intracellular folate concentrations. Specifically, low folate concentrations ensure a greater competition for 5,10-methylenetetrahydrofolate, favoring one-carbon commitment to thymidylate synthesis and formyl-folate reactions rather than 5-methyl-tetrahdyrofolate synthesis.[46,369,370] Low folate concentrations, thus, may mimic the MTHFR 677TT genotype and may explain why subjects with the wild type enzyme have better hearing when folate levels are low. If our findings are confirmed in other (larger) populations, then more research should be conducted on how folate status affects the formyl-folate / methyl-folate ratio and the possible importance of methenyl and formyl-folate reactions in relation to neurodegenerative disorders. How can we explain that only the relation between folate and hearing depends on genotype, and not cognitive function? A possible explanation may the sensitivity of the cochlea to perturbations in both mitochondria and folate metabolism.

Sensorineural hearing loss, the pattern of hearing loss characterizing age-related hearing loss, is the first symptom seen in patients with mitochondrial disorders, before other neurodegenerative processes and cardiomyopathy take place.[371] In addition sensorineural hearing loss is a common side effect of folate analogue therapy used mainly against cancers, appearing within days after therapy commencement.[372] Deterioration of hearing in the ultra high frequencies may take place even sooner.[373] Several lines of evidence suggest that mitochondrial function and folate metabolism are interrelated. Folate analogue-induced cytotoxicity is thought to be due to the inhibition of complexes I and IV of the electron transport chain located in the mitochondria.[374] Indeed, sensitivity to folate analogue therapy is dependent on the involvement of mitochondria as shown from *in vitro* studies using Chinese hamster ovary cells with selective expression of folypolyglutamate synthetase, an enzyme responsible for folate sequestration, located in the mitochondria and cytosol.[375] As a consequence of folate analogue therapy, folate content decreased seven-fold and three-fold in the mitochondria and cytosol, respectively in those studies.[375] Thus, the mitochondria are responsible for a drastic drop in folate levels subsequent to folate analogue therapy, considering that approximately half of cellular folate is located in mitochondria.[46] As mentioned earlier, 10-

formyltetrahydrofolate was able to increase oxidative phosphorylation;[260] results from previous studies suggest that treatment with mitochondrial metabolites which improve oxidative phosphorylation also improve hearing and cognitive function.[287,368] Clearly, sensorineural hearing loss is easily affected by mitochondrial disorders or anomalies in folate metabolism, however, whether 10-formyltetrahydrofolate also acts as a mitochondrial metabolite that improves hearing requires further research.

To test the hypothesis that DNA infidelity and mitochondrial decay are involved in age-related neurodegenerative disorders, such as cognitive decline and age-related hearing loss, we need trials to investigate the effect of mitochondrial metabolites (e.g. coenzyme Q_{10}, α-lipoic acid, melatonin and acetyl L-carnitine), both in the short-term and long-term, on hearing levels and cognitive performance. To support or refute or hypotheses, large cohorts need to examine polymorphisms in genes encoding folate-related enzymes, including the MTHFR C677T and MTHFR A1298C, and other polymorphisms which are involved in DNA fidelity and general folate status, such as the double (2R2R) or triple (3R3R) tandem repeat in the promoter region of thymidylate synthase and cytosolic serine hydroxymethyltransferase C1420T, respectively (See Figure 1.1). Finally, more *in vitro* and *in vivo* studies need to be conducted which examine the effect of greater one-carbon commitment to *de novo* nucleotide synthesis and 10-formyltetrahydrofolate synthesis on the mitochondria and DNA stability.

Conclusion

Increased concentrations of folate, independent of its role in homocysteine-lowering, are weakly associated with decreased risk of cardiovascular disease and better cognitive function, but not with hearing acuity. Inflammation, as measured by oxidized LDL, autoantibodies against oxidized LDL, C-reactive protein and soluble intercellular adhesion molecule-1, is not likely to be an immediate factor to explain the link between folate and health, as these markers were immune to one-year folic acid supplementation. We speculated that phenotypic differences related to MTHFR 677C→T genotype, other than hyperhomocysteinemia, may be important perhaps through conserving DNA fidelity and mitochondrial bioenergetic efficiency.

Further research is required to explore the role of folate in these conditions, as well as to justify health claims of folate. If faced with the decision whether to fortify the national food chain with folic acid, public health policy makers should wait for the large trials to report their findings on the effects of folic acid, alone or in combination with other B vitamins, on cardiovascular disease and dementia. In 2005, the FACIT trial researchers will report their findings on the effect of three-year folic acid supplementation on cardiovascular disease risk, cognitive decline and age-related hearing loss.

References

1. Smith R. "Let food be thy medicine....". *Br Med J* 2004;(7433)328:0.

2. Mintz SW. Time, sugar and sweetness. *Marx Perspect* 1979;2:56-73.

3. Hoffbrand AV, Weir DG. The history of folic acid. *Br J Haematol* 2001;113:579-589.

4. Lucock M. Is folic acid the ultimate functional food component for disease prevention? *Br Med J* 2004;328:211-214.

5. Blom HJ. Diseases and drugs associated with hyperhomocysteinemia. In: Carmel R, Jacobsen DW, eds. *Homocysteine in health and disease.* Cambridge: Cambridge University Press, 2001:331-340.

6. Health Council of The Netherlands. *Dietary reference intakes: vitamin B_6, folate and vitamin B_{12}.* 2003.

7. Venn BJ, Mann JI, Williams SM, et al. Dietary counseling to increase natural folate intake: a randomized, placebo-controlled trial in free-living subjects to assess effects on serum folate and plasma total homocysteine. *Am J Clin Nutr* 2002;76:758-765.

8. Riddell LJ, Chisholm A, Williams S, Mann JI. Dietary strategies for lowering homocysteine concentrations. *Am J Clin Nutr* 2000;71:1448-1454.

9. Broekmans WMR, Klöpping-Ketelaars IAA, Schuurman CRWC, et al. Fruits and vegetables increase plasma carotenoids and vitamins and decrease homocysteine in humans. *J Nutr* 2000;130:1578-1583.

10. Brouwer IA, van Dusseldorp M, West CE, et al. Dietary folate from vegetables and citrus fruit decreases plasma homocysteine concentrations in humans in a dietary controlled trial. *J Nutr* 1999;129:1135-1139.

11. Appel LJ, Miller ER, Jee SH, et al. Effect of dietary patterns on serum homocysteine: results of a randomized, controlled feeding study. *Circulation* 2000;102:852-857.

12. van Dam RM, Grievink L, Ocké MC, Feskens EJM. Patterns of food consumption and risk factors for cardiovascular disease in the general Dutch population. *Am J Clin Nutr* 2003;77:1156-1163.

13. Kerver JM, Yang EJ, Bianchi L, Song WO. Dietary patterns associated with risk factors for cardiovascular disease in healthy US adults. *Am J Clin Nutr* 2003;78:1103-1110.

14. Steffen LM, Jacobs D-RJ, Stevens J, Shahar E, Carithers T, Folsom AR. Associations of whole-grain, refined-grain, and fruit and vegetable consumption with risks of all-cause mortality and incident coronary artery disease and ischemic stroke: the Atherosclerosis Risk in Communities (ARIC) Study. *Am J Clin Nutr* 2003;78:383-390.

15. Hu FB. Plant-based foods and prevention of cardiovascular disease: an overview. *Am J Clin Nutr* 2003;78:544S-551S.

16. Gao X, Bermudez OI, Tucker KL. Plasma C-reactive protein and homocysteine concentrations are related to frequent fruit and vegetable intake in Hispanic and non-Hispanic white elders. *J Nutr* 2004;134:913-918.

17. Gao X, Yao M, McCrory MA, et al. Dietary pattern is associated with homocysteine and B vitamin status in an urban Chinese population. *J Nutr* 2003;133:3636-3642.

18. Barzi F, Woodward M, Marfisi RM, et al. Mediterranean diet and all-causes mortality after myocardial infarction: results from the GISSI-Prevenzione trial. *Eur J Clin Nutr* 2003;57:604-611.

19. Lökk J. News and views on folate and elderly persons. *J Gerontol A Biol Sci Med Sci* 2003;58:354-361.

20. Clarke R, Grimley Evans J, Schneede J, et al. Vitamin B12 and folate deficiency in later life. *Age Ageing* 2004;33:34-41.

21. Bolander-Gouaille, C. *Focus on Homocysteine and the Vitamins Involved in its Metabolism.* 2, 69-117. 2002. France, Springer Verlag.

22. Stover PJ, Garza C. Bringing individuality to public health recommendations. *J Nutr* 2002;132:2476S-2480S.

23. Medical Research Council. Prevention of neural tube defects: results of the Medical Research Council Vitamin Study. MRC Vitamin Study Research Group. *Lancet* 1991;338:131-137.

24. De Wals P, Rusen ID, Lee NS, Morin P, Niyonsenga T. Trend in prevalence of neural tube defects in Quebec. *Birth Defects Res Part A Clin Mol Teratol* 2003;67:919-923.

25. Yang Q, Friedman JM, Botto LD. Improvement in cardiovascular and stroke mortality after flour fortification with folic acid in the United States. Abstract for the

Late Breaking Science Program, 44th Annual Conference on Cardiovascular Disease Epidemiology and Prevention, 3-6 March 2004, San Francisco, California USA.

26. Mills JL, Von Kohorn I, Conley MR, et al. Low vitamin B-12 concentrations in patients without anemia: the effect of folic acid fortification of grain. *Am J Clin Nutr* 2003;77:1474-1477.

27. Health Council of The Netherlands. *Risks of folic acid fortification.* 2000.

28. Windham GC, Shaw GM, Todoroff K, Swan SH. Miscarriage and use of multi-vitamins or folic acid. *Am J Med Genet* 2000;90:261-262.

29. Hook EB. Folic acid: abortifacient or pseudoabortifacient? *Am J Med Genet* 2000;92:301-302.

30. Munoz-Moran E, Dieguez-Lucena JL, Fernandez-Arcas N, Peran-Mesa S, Reyes-Engel A. Genetic selection and folate intake during pregnancy. *Lancet* 1998;352:1120-1121.

31. Kim Y-I. Role of folate in colon cancer development and progression. *J Nutr* 2003;133:3731S-3739S.

32. the Homocysteine Studies Collaboration. Homocysteine and risk of ischemic heart disease and stroke - A meta-analysis. *J Am Med Assoc* 2002;288:2015-2022.

33. Oakley GP. Delaying folic acid fortification of flour. *Br Med J* 2002;324:1348-1349.

34. Rimm EB, Willett WC, Hu FB, et al. Folate and vitamin B_6 from diet and supplements in relation to risk of coronary heart disease among women. *J Am Med Assoc* 1998;279:359-364.

35. Magni E, Bianchetti A, Rozzini R, Trabucchi M. Influence of nutritional intake on 6-year mortality in an Italian elderly population. *J Nutr Elder* 1994;13:25-34.

36. Voutilainen S, Rissanen TH, Virtanen J, Lakka TA, Salonen JT. Low dietary folate intake is associated with an excess incidence of acute coronary events: the Kuopio Ischemic Heart Disease Risk Factor Study. *Circulation* 2001;103:2674-2680.

37. Folsom AR, Nieto FJ, McGovern PG, et al. Prospective study of coronary heart disease incidence in relation to fasting total homocysteine, related genetic polymorphisms, and B vitamins: the Atherosclerosis Risk in Communities (ARIC) study. *Circulation* 1998;98:204-210.

38. Chasan-Taber L, Selhub J, Rosenberg IH, et al. A prospective study of folate and vitamin B_6 and risk of myocardial infarction in US physicians. *J Am Coll Nutr* 1996;15:136-143.

39. de Bree A, Verschuren WMM, Bjørke-Monsen A-L, et al. Effect of the methylenetetrahydrofolate reductase 677C→T mutation on the relations among folate intake and plasma folate and homocysteine concentrations in a general population sample. *Am J Clin Nutr* 2003;77:687-693.

40. Hung J, Beilby JP, Knuiman MW, Divitini M. Folate and vitamin B-12 and risk of fatal cardiovascular disease: cohort study from Busselton, Western Australia. *Br Med J* 2003;326:131-134.

41. Morrison HI, Schaubel D, Desmeules M, Wigle DT. Serum folate and risk of fatal coronary heart disease. *J Am Med Assoc* 1996;275:1893-1896.

42. Loria CM, Ingram DD, Feldman JJ, Wright JD, Madans JH. Serum folate and cardiovascular disease mortality among US men and women. *Arch Intern Med* 2000;160:3258-3262.

43. Ford ES, Byers TE, Giles WH. Serum folate and chronic disease risk: findings from a cohort of United States adults. *Int J Epidemiol* 1998;27:592-598.

44. Giles WH, Kittner SJ, Anda RF, Croft JB, Casper ML. Serum folate and risk for ischemic stroke. First National Health and Nutrition Examination Survey epidemiologic follow-up study. *Stroke* 1995;26:1166-1170.

45. Voutilainen S, Lakka TA, Porkkala-Sarataho E, Rissanen T, Kaplan GA, Salonen JT. Low serum folate concentrations are associated with an excess incidence of acute coronary events: the Kuopio Ischaemic Heart Disease Risk Factor Study. *Eur J Clin Nutr* 2000;54:424-428.

46. Suh JR, Herbig AK, Stover PJ. New perspectives on folate catabolism. *Annu Rev Nutr* 2001;21:255-282.

47. Toole JF, Malinow MR, Chambless LE, et al. Lowering homocysteine in patients with ischemic stroke to prevent recurrent stroke, myocardial infarction, and death: the Vitamin Intervention for Stroke Prevention (VISP) randomized controlled trial. *J Am Med Assoc* 2004;291:565-575.

48. Durga J, Schouten EG, Bots ML, et al. Design of a randomized controlled trial of the effect of folic acid on atherosclerosis and cognitive function. Abstract for the 3rd International Conference of Homocysteine Metabolism, 1-5 July 2001, Sorrento Italy.

49. Wald NJ, Law MR. A strategy to reduce cardiovascular disease by more than 80%. *Br Med J* 2003;326:1419.

50. Wald DS, Law M, Morris JK. Homocysteine and cardiovascular disease: evidence on causality from a meta-analysis. BMJ 2002;325:1202.

51. United States Food and Drug Administration. Settlement reached for health claim relating B vitamins and vascular disease. http://www.cfsan.fda.gov/~dms/ds-hclbv.html (last accessed June 2004).

52. Schnyder G, Roffi M, Pin R, et al. Decreased rate of coronary restenosis after lowering of plasma homocysteine levels. *N Engl J Med* 2001;345:1593-1600.

53. Lange H, Suryapranata H, De Luca G, et al. Folate therapy and in-stent restenosis after coronary stenting. *N Engl J Med* 2004;350:2673-2681.

54. Till U, Jentsch A, Röhl P, et al. In patients at risk to cerebral ischemia an oral substitution with vitamin B6, B12 and folic acid leads to a significant decrease of the intima/media-thickness of the carotids - results of a randomised, placebo-controlled trial. *J Inherit Metab Dis* 2003;26(Suppl.1):13.

55. Marcucci R, Zanazzi M, Bertoni E, et al. Vitamin supplementation reduces the progression of atherosclerosis in hyperhomocysteinemic renal-transplant recipients. *Transplantation* 2003;75:1551-1555.

56. Vermeulen EGJ, Stehouwer CDA, Twisk JWR, et al. Effect of homocysteine-lowering treatment with folic acid plus vitamin B_6 on progression of subclinical atherosclerosis: a randomised, placebo-controlled trial. *Lancet* 2000;355:517-522.

57. Bots ML, Dijk JM, Oren A, Grobbee DE. Carotid intima-media thickness, arterial stiffness and risk of cardiovascular disease: current evidence. *J Hypertens* 2002;20:2317-2325.

58. Bostom AG, Garber C. Endpoints for homocysteine-lowering trials. *Lancet* 2000;355:511-512.

59. Baker F, Picton D, Blackwood S, et al. Blinded comparison of folic acid and placebo in patients with ischemic heart disease: an outcome trial. Circulation 2002;106(Suppl. II):II-741.

60. de Jong SC, Stehouwer CDA, van den-Berg M, Geurts TW, Bouter LM, Rauwerda JA. Normohomocysteinaemia and vitamin-treated hyperhomocysteinaemia are associated with similar risks of cardiovascular events in patients with premature peripheral arterial occlusive disease. A prospective cohort study. *J Intern Med* 1999;246:87-96.

61. Vermeulen EGJ, Rauwerda JA, Erix P, et al. Normohomocysteinaemia and vitamin-treated hyperhomocysteinaemia are associated with similar risks of cardiovascular events in patients with premature atherothrombotic cerebrovascular disease. A prospective cohort study. *Neth J Med* 2000;56:138-146.

62. Hackam DG, Peterson JC, Spence JD. What level of plasma homocyst(e)ine should be treated? Effects of vitamin therapy on progression of carotid atherosclerosis in patients with homocyst(e)ine levels above and below 14 μmol/L. *Am J Hypertens* 2000;13:105-110.

63. Peterson JC, Spence JD. Vitamins and progression of atherosclerosis in hyper-homocyst(e)inaemia. *Lancet* 1998;351:263.

64. Liem AH, van Boven AJ, Veeger NJGM, et al. Efficacy of folic acid when added to statin therapy in patients with hypercholesterolemia following acute myocardial infarction: a randomised pilot trial. *Int J Cardiol* 2004;93:175-179.

65. Liem A, Reynierse-Buitenwerf GH, Zwinderman AH, Jukema JW, van Veldhuisen DJ. Secondary prevention with folic acid: effects on clinical outcomes. *J Am Coll Cardiol* 2003;41:2105-2113.

66. Schnyder G, Roffi M, Flammer Y, et al. Effect of homocysteine-lowering therapy on restenosis after percutaneous coronary intervention for narrowings in small coronary arteries. *Am J Cardiol* 2003;91:1265-1269.

67. Schnyder G, Roffi M, Flammer Y, Pin R, Hess OM. Effect of homocysteine-lowering therapy with folic acid, vitamin B_{12}, vitamin B_6 on clinical outcome after percutaneous coronary intervention: the Swiss Heart study: a randomized controlled trial. *J Am Med Assoc* 2002;288:973-979.

68. Wrone EM, Hornberger JM, Zehnder JL, McCann LM, Coplon NS, Fortmann SP. Randomized trial of folic acid for prevention of cardiovascular events in end-stage renal disease. *J Am Soc Nephrol* 2004;15:420-426.

69. Vermeulen EGJ, Stehouwer CDA, Valk J, et al. Effect of homocysteine-lowering treatment with folic acid plus vitamin B on cerebrovascular atherosclerosis and white matter abnormalities as determined by MRA and MRI: a placebo-controlled, randomized trial. *Eur J Clin Invest* 2004;34:256-261.

70. Jacques PF, Tucker KL. Are dietary patterns useful for understanding the role of diet in chronic disease? *Am J Clin Nutr* 2001;73:1-2.

71. Nurk E, Tell GS, Vollset SE, et al. Changes in lifestyle and plasma total homocysteine: the Hordaland Homocysteine Study. *Am J Clin Nutr* 2004;79:812-819.

72. Fung TT, Rimm EB, Spiegelman D, et al. Association between dietary patterns and plasma biomarkers of obesity and cardiovascular disease risk. *Am J Clin Nutr* 2001;73:61-67.

73. Fung TT, Willett WC, Stampfer MJ, Manson JE, Hu FB. Dietary patterns and the risk of coronary heart disease in women. *Arch Intern Med* 2001;161:1857-1862.

74. Clarke R. Commentary: An updated review of the published studies of homocysteine and cardiovascular disease. *Int J Epidemiol* 2002;31:70-71.

75. de Bree A, Verschuren WMM, Kromhout D, Mennen LI, Blom HJ. Homocysteine and coronary heart disease: the importance of a distinction between low and high risk subjects. *Int J Epidemiol* 2002;31:1268-1272.

76. Brennan P. Commentary: Mendelian randomization and gene-environment interaction. *Int J Epidemiol* 2004;33:17-21.

77. Davey Smith G, Ebrahim S. 'Mendelian randomization': can genetic epidemiology contribute to understanding environmental determinants of disease? *Int J Epidemiol* 2003;32:1-22.

78. Klerk M, Verhoef P, Clarke R, et al. MTHFR 677C→T polymorphism and risk of coronary heart disease: a meta-analysis. *J Am Med Assoc* 2002;288:2023-2031.

79. Keavney B. Commentary: Katan's remarkable foresight: genes and causality 18 years on. *Int J Epidemiol* 2004;33:11-14.

80. Davey Smith G, Ebrahim S. Mendelian randomization: prospects, potentials, and limitations. *Int J Epidemiol* 2004;33:30-42.

81. Vivekananthan DP, Penn MS, Sapp SK, Hsu A, Topol EJ. Use of antioxidant vitamins for the prevention of cardiovascular disease: meta-analysis of randomised trials. *Lancet* 2003;361:2017-2023.

82. Jacobs DRJ, Steffen LM. Nutrients, foods, and dietary patterns as exposures in research: a framework for food synergy. *Am J Clin Nutr* 2003;78:508S-513S.

83. Hu FB, Willett WC. Optimal diets for prevention of coronary heart disease. *J Am Med Assoc* 2002;288:2569-2578.

84. Nestel PJ, Chronopoulos A, Cehun M. Arterial stiffness is rapidly induced by raising the plasma homocysteine concentration with methionine. *Atherosclerosis* 2003;171:83-86.

85. de Bree A, Mennen LI, Bertrais S, et al. Relation between homocysteine concentrations and structural and functional arterial parameters in a French general population. *J Inherit Metab Dis* 2003;26 (Suppl.1):24.

86. Smilde TJ, van den Berkmortel FWPJ, Boers GHJ, et al. Carotid and femoral artery wall thickness and stiffness in patients at risk for cardiovascular disease, with special emphasis on hyperhomocysteinemia. *Arterioscler Thromb Vasc Biol* 1998;18:1958-1963.

87. Lambert J, van den Berg M, Steyn M, Rauwerda JA, Donker AJM, Stehouwer CDA. Familial hyperhomocysteinaemia and endothelium-dependent vasodilatation and arterial distensibility of large arteries. *Cardiovasc Res* 1999;42:743-751.

88. Bortolotto LA, Safar ME, Billaud E, et al. Plasma homocysteine, aortic stiffness, and renal function in hypertensive patients. *Hypertension* 1999;34:837-842.

89. van Dijk RAJM, Rauwerda JA, Steyn M, Twisk JWR, Stehouwer CDA. Long-term homocysteine-lowering treatment with folic acid plus pyridoxine is associated with decreased blood pressure but not with improved brachial artery endothelium-dependent vasodilation or carotid artery stiffness - A 2-year, randomized, placebo-controlled trial. *Arterioscler Thromb Vasc Biol* 2001;21:2072-2079.

90. Mangoni AA, Sherwood RA, Swift CG, Jackson SHD. Folic acid enhances endothelial function and reduces blood pressure in smokers: a randomized controlled trial. *J Intern Med* 2002;252:497-503.

91. van Guldener C, Lambert J, ter Wee PM, Donker AJM, Stehouwer CDA. Carotid artery stiffness in patients with end-stage renal disease: no effect of long-term homocysteine-lowering therapy. *Clin Nephrol* 2000;53:33-41.

92. Calvaresi E, Bryan J. B vitamins, cognition, and aging: a review. *J Gerontol B Psychol Sci Soc Sci* 2001;56:327-339.

93. Selhub J, Bagley LC, Miller J, Rosenberg IH. B vitamins, homocysteine, and neurocognitive function in the elderly. *Am J Clin Nutr* 2000;71:614S-620S.

94. Malouf M, Grimley EJ, Areosa SA. Folic acid with or without vitamin B12 for cognition and dementia. *Cochrane Database Syst Rev* 2003;CD004514.

95. Rapin JR, Le Poncin M, Grebyl J. Blood folates deficiencies and cognitive functions in aging. *Trends Biomed.Gerontol* 1988;1:221-223.

96. Heseker H, Kübler W, Pudel V, Westenhöfer J. Interaction of vitamins with mental performance. *Bibl Nutr Dieta* 1995;43-55.

97. Fioravanti M, Ferrario E, Massaia M, et al. Low folate levels in the cognitive decline of elderly patients and the efficacy of folate as a treatment for improving memory deficits. *Arch Gerontol Geriatr* 1997;26:1-13.

98. Nilsson K, Gustafson L, Hultberg B. Improvement of cognitive functions after cobalamin/folate supplementation in elderly patients with dementia and elevated plasma homocysteine. *Int J Geriatr Psychiatry* 2001;16:609-614.

99. Bryan J, Calvaresi E, Hughes D. Short-term folate, vitamin B-12 or vitamin B-6 supplementation slightly affects memory performance but not mood in women of various ages. *J Nutr* 2002;132:1345-1356.

100. Clarke R, Harrison G, Richards S, on behalf of the VITAL trial collaborative group. Effect of vitamins and aspirin on markers of platelet activation, oxidative stress and homocysteine in people at high risk of dementia. *J Intern Med* 2003;254:67-75.

101. van Boxtel MPJ, Buntinx F, Houx PJ, Metsemakers JF, Knottnerus A, Jolles J. The relation between morbidity and cognitive performance in a normal aging population. *J Gerontol A Biol Sci Med Sci* 1998;53:M147-M154.

102. Houston DK, Johnson MA, Nozza RJ, et al. Age-related hearing loss, vitamin B-12, and folate in elderly women. *Am J Clin Nutr* 1999;69:564-571.

103. Berner B, Ødum L, Parving A. Age-related hearing impairment and B vitamin status. *Acta Oto-Laryngol* 2000;120:633-637.

104. Faraci FM. Hyperhomocysteinemia: a million ways to lose control. *Arterioscler Thromb Vasc Biol* 2003;23:371-373.

105. Doshi SN, McDowell IFW, Moat SJ, et al. Folate improves endothelial function in coronary artery disease: an effect mediated by reduction of intracellular superoxide? *Arterioscler Thromb Vasc Biol* 2001;21:1196-1202.

106. Moat SJ, Hill MH, McDowell IFW, et al. Reduction in plasma total homocysteine through increasing folate intake in healthy individuals is not associated with changes in measures of antioxidant activity or oxidant damage. *Eur J Clin Nutr* 2003;57:483-489.

107. Woodside JV, Young IS, Yarnell JW, et al. Antioxidants, but not B-group vitamins increase the resistance of low-density lipoprotein to oxidation: a randomized, factorial design, placebo-controlled trial. *Atherosclerosis* 1999;144:419-427.

108. Doshi SN, McDowell IFW, Moat SJ, et al. Folic acid improves endothelial function in coronary artery disease via mechanisms largely independent of homocysteine lowering. *Circulation* 2002;105:22-26.

109. Klerk M. The effect of folic acid supplementation for 1 year on hemostasis markers in healthy elderly. In: *Homocysteine and coronary heart disease; the role of polymorphic genes and hemostasis.* Ph.D. Thesis Wageningen University. Wageningen: Klerk M, 2002:87-103.

110. Vermeulen EGJ, Rauwerda JA, van den Berg M, et al. Homocysteine-lowering treatment with folic acid plus vitamin B6 lowers urinary albumin excretion but not plasma markers of endothelial function or C-reactive protein: further analysis of secondary end-points of a randomized clinical trial. *Eur J Clin Invest* 2003;33:209-215.

111. Ford ES, Smith SJ, Stroup DF, Steinberg KK, Mueller PW, Thacker SB. Homocyst(e)ine and cardiovascular disease: a systematic review of the evidence with special emphasis on case-control studies and nested case-control studies. *Int J Epidemiol* 2002;31:59-70.

112. Brattström L, Wilcken DEL. Homocysteine and cardiovascular disease: cause or effect? *Am J Clin Nutr* 2000;72:315-323.

113. van Aken BE, Dekkers PEP, Pajkrt D, et al. Hyperhomocysteinemia in experimental endotoxemia in humans. In: *Inflammation markers, vascular disease and homocysteine*. Ph.D. Thesis University of Amsterdam. Amsterdam: van Aken BE, 1999;115-123.

114. Selhub J. Homocysteine metabolism. *Annu Rev Nutr* 1999;19:217-246.

115. Homocysteine Lowering Trialists' Collaboration. Lowering blood homocysteine with folic acid based supplements: meta-analysis of randomised trials. *Br Med J* 1998;316:894-898.

116. Espeland MA, Hoen H, Byington R, Howard G, Riley WA, Furberg CD. Spatial distribution of carotid intimal-medial thickness as measured by B-mode ultrasonography. *Stroke* 1994;25:1812-1819.

117. Bots ML, de Jong PTVM, Hofman A, Grobbee DE. Left, right, near or far wall common carotid intima-media thickness measurements: associations with cardiovascular disease and lower extremity arterial atherosclerosis. *J Clin Epidemiol* 1997;50:801-807.

118. Demuth K, Drunat S, Girerd X, et al. Homocysteine is the only plasma thiol associated with carotid artery remodeling. *Atherosclerosis* 2002;165:167-174.

119. Folsom AR, Nieto FJ, Sorlie P, Chambless LE, Graham DY. *Helicobacter pylori* seropositivity and coronary heart disease incidence. Atherosclerosis Risk In Communities (ARIC) Study Investigators. *Circulation* 1998;98:845-850.

120. Mazza A, Motti C, Nulli A, et al. Serum homocysteine, MTHFR gene polymorphism, and carotid intimal-medial thickness in NIDDM subjects. *J Thromb Thrombolysis* 1999;8:207-212.

121. Suwelack B, Gerhardt U, Witta J, Hohage H. Total serum homocysteine does not influence carotid intimal media thickness. *Transplant Proc* 2001;33:2381-2383.

122. Anand SS, Yusuf S, Vuksan V, et al. Differences in risk factors, atherosclerosis, and cardiovascular disease between ethnic groups in Canada: the Study of Health Assessment and Risk in Ethnic groups (SHARE). *Lancet* 2000;356:279-284.

123. McCully KS. Vascular pathology of homocysteinemia: implications for the pathogenesis of arteriosclerosis. *Am J Pathol* 1969;56:111-128.

124. Yap S, Boers GHJ, Wilcken B, et al. Vascular outcome in patients with homocystinuria due to cystathionine β-synthase deficiency treated chronically: a multicenter observational study. Arterioscler.Thromb.Vasc.Biol. 2001;21:2080-2085.

125. Megnien JL, Gariepy J, Saudubray JM, et al. Evidence of carotid artery wall hypertrophy in homozygous homocystinuria. *Circulation* 1998;98:2276-2281.

126. de Valk HW, van Eeden MK, Banga JD, et al. Evaluation of the presence of premature atherosclerosis in adults with heterozygosity for cystathionine-β-synthase deficiency. *Stroke* 1996;27:1134-1136.

127. Clarke R, Fitzgerald D, O'Brien C, et al. Hyperhomocysteinaemia: a risk factor for extracranial carotid artery atherosclerosis. *Ir J Med Sci* 1992;161:61-65.

128. Rubba P, Faccenda F, Pauciullo P, et al. Early signs of vascular disease in homocystinuria: a noninvasive study by ultrasound methods in eight families with cystathionine-β-synthase deficiency. *Metabolism* 1990;39:1191-1195.

129. Rubba P, Mercuri M, Faccenda F, et al. Premature carotid atherosclerosis: does it occur in both familial hypercholesterolemia and homocystinuria? Ultrasound assessment of arterial intima-media thickness and blood flow velocity. *Stroke* 1994;25:943-950.

130. Oh J, Wunsch R, Turzer M, et al. Advanced coronary and carotid arteriopathy in young adults with childhood-onset chronic renal failure. *Circulation* 2002;106:100-105.

131. Kennedy R, Case C, Fathi R, Johnson D, Isbel N, Marwick TH. Does renal failure cause an atherosclerotic milieu in patients with end-stage renal disease? *Am J Med* 2001;110:198-204.

132. Lim PS, Hung WR, Wei YH. Polymorphism in methylenetetrahydrofolate reductase gene: Its impact on plasma homocysteine levels and carotid atherosclerosis in ESRD patients receiving hemodialysis. *Nephron* 2001;87:249-256.

133. Libetta C, Villa G, Pirrelli S, et al. Homocysteine plasma levels correlate with intimal carotid artery thickness in haemodialysis patients. *Nephrol Dial Transplant* 2001;16:2444-2445.

134. Maeda N, Sawayama Y, Tatsukawa M, et al. Carotid artery lesions and atherosclerotic risk factors in Japanese hemodialysis patients. *Atherosclerosis* 2003;169:183-192.

135. Haraki T, Takegoshi T, Kitoh C, et al. Hyperhomocysteinemia, diabetes mellitus, and carotid atherosclerosis independently increase atherosclerotic vascular disease outcome in Japanese patients with end-stage renal disease. *Clin Nephrol* 2001;56:132-139.

136. Brzósko S, Łebkowska U, Małyszko J, Hryszko T, Pawlak K, Myśliwiec M. Correlation between carotid intima-media thickness and hematocrit and hemoglobin values in renal transplant recipients. *Clin Transplant* 2001;15:349-353.

137. Suwelack B, Gerhardt U, Witta J, Rahn KH, Hohage H. Effect of homocysteine on carotid intima-media thickness after renal transplantation. *Clin Transplant* 2000;14:555-560.

138. Zoungas S, Ristevski S, Lightfoot P, et al. Proceedings of the High Blood Pressure Research Council of Australia - Carotid artery intima-medial thickness is increased in chronic renal failure. *Clin Exp Pharmacol Physiol* 2000;27:639-641.

139. Ohkuma T, Minagawa T, Takada N, Ohno M, Oda H, Ohashi H. C-reactive protein, lipoprotein(a), homocysteine, and male sex contribute to carotid atherosclerosis in peritoneal dialysis patients. *Am J Kidney Dis* 2003;42:355-361.

140. Pannier B, Guerin AP, Marchais SJ, Metivier F, Safar ME, London GM. Postischemic vasodilation, endothelial activation, and cardiovascular remodeling in end-stage renal disease. *Kidney Int* 2000;57:1091-1099.

141. Sakurabayashi T, Fujimoto M, Takaesu Y, et al. Association between plasma homocysteine concentration and carotid atherosclerosis in hemodialysis patients. *Jpn Circ J* 1999;63:692-696.

142. Hopkins PN, Stephenson S, Wu LL, Riley WA, Xin YP, Hunt SC. Evaluation of coronary risk factors in patients with heterozygous familial hypercholesterolemia. *Am J Cardiol* 2001;87:547-553.

143. Raal FJ, Pilcher GJ, Waisberg R, Buthelezi EP, Veller MG, Joffe BI. Low-density lipoprotein cholesterol bulk is the pivotal determinant of atherosclerosis in familial hypercholesterolemia. *Am J Cardiol* 1999;83:1330-1333.

144. Tonstad S, Joakimsen O, Stensland-Bugge E, et al. Risk factors related to carotid intima-media thickness and plaque in children with familial hypercholesterolemia and control subjects. *Arterioscler Thromb Vasc Biol* 1996;16:984-991.

145. Voutilainen S, Alfthan G, Nyyssönen K, Salonen R, Salonen JT. Association between elevated plasma total homocysteine and increased common carotid artery wall thickness. *Ann Med* 1998;30:300-306.

146. Scaglione L, Gambino R, Rolfo E, et al. Plasma homocysteine, methylenetetrahydrofolate reductase gene polymorphism and carotid intima-media thickness in Italian type 2 diabetic patients. *Eur J Clin Invest* 2002;32:24-28.

147. Mazza A, Motti C, Nulli A, et al. Lack of association between carotid intima-media thickness and methylenetetrahydrofolate reductase gene polymorphism or serum homocysteine in non-insulin-dependent diabetes mellitus. *Metabolism* 2000;49:718-723.

148. Fagerberg B, Wallenfeldt K, Alenhag E-L, Bokemark L, Wikstrand J. High-normal serum homocysteine concentrations are associated with an increased risk of early atherosclerotic carotid artery wall lesions. *J Hypertens* 2000;18:1523-1525.

149. Becker A, Henry RMA, Kostense PJ, et al. Plasma homocysteine and *S*-adenosylmethionine in erythrocytes as determinants of carotid intima-media thickness: different effects in diabetic and non-diabetic individuals. The Hoorn Study. *Atherosclerosis* 2003;169:323-330.

150. Mercié P, Thiébaut R, Lavignolle V, et al. Evaluation of cardiovascular risk factors in HIV-1 infected patients using carotid intima-media thickness measurement. *Ann Med* 2002;34:55-63.

151. Ames PRJ, Margarita A, Delgado Alves J, Tommasino C, Iannaccone L, Brancaccio V. Anticardiolipin antibody titre and plasma homocysteine level independently predict intima media thickness of carotid arteries in subjects with idiopathic antiphospholipid antibodies. *Lupus* 2002;11:208-214.

152. Svenungsson E, Jensen-Urstad K, Heimbürger M, et al. Risk factors for cardio-vascular disease in systemic lupus erythematosus. *Circulation* 2001;104:1887-1893.

153. Nakaso K, Yasui K, Kowa H, et al. Hypertrophy of IMC of carotid artery in Parkinson's disease is associated with L-DOPA, homocysteine, and MTHFR genotype. *J Neurol Sci* 2003;207:19-23.

154. Magyar MT, Szikszai Z, Balla J, et al. Early-onset carotid atherosclerosis is associated with increased intima-media thickness and elevated serum levels of inflammatory markers. *Stroke* 2003;34:58-63.

155. Kawamoto R, Doi T, Tokunaga H. Association of plasma homocysteine concentrations with carotid atherosclerosis in elderly Japanese. *Intern Med* 2001;40:1189-1194.

156. Tsai MY, Arnett DK, Eckfeldt JH, Williams RR, Ellison RC. Plasma homocysteine and its association with carotid intimal-medial wall thickness and prevalent coronary heart disease: NHLBI Family Heart Study. *Atherosclerosis* 2000;151:519-524.

157. Lupattelli G, Rufini S, Locati EH, et al. Hyperhomocyst(e)inemia is associated with carotid atherosclerosis. *Angiology* 1999;50:823-830.

158. Okamura T, Kitamura A, Moriyama Y, et al. Plasma level of homocysteine is correlated to extracranial carotid-artery atherosclerosis in non-hypertensive Japanese. *J Cardiovasc Risk* 1999;6:371-377.

159. Rohde LE, Lee RT, Rivero J, et al. Circulating cell adhesion molecules are correlated with ultrasound-based assessment of carotid atherosclerosis. *Arterioscler Thromb Vasc Biol* 1998;18:1765-1770.

160. Demuth K, Moatti N, Hanon O, Benoit MO, Safar M, Girerd X. Opposite effects of plasma homocysteine and the methylenetetrahydrofolate reductase C677T mutation on carotid artery geometry in asymptomatic adults. *Arterioscler Thromb Vasc Biol* 1998;18:1838-1843.

161. Noto R, Neri S, Molino G, et al. Hyperhomocysteinemia in menopausal hypertension: an added risk factor and a dangerous association for organ damage. *Eur Rev Med Pharmacol Sci* 2002;6:81-87.

162. Adachi H, Hirai Y, Fujiura Y, Matsuoka H, Satoh A, Imaizumi T. Plasma homocysteine levels and atherosclerosis in Japan - Epidemiological study by use of carotid ultrasonography. *Stroke* 2002;33:2177-2181.

163. McQuillan BM, Beilby JP, Nidorf M, Thompson PL, Hung J. Hyperhomocysteinemia but not the C677T mutation of methylenetetrahydrofolate reductase is an independent risk determinant of carotid wall thickening. The Perth Carotid Ultrasound Disease Assessment Study (CUDAS). *Circulation* 1999;99:2383-2388.

164. Malinow MR, Nieto FJ, Szklo M, Chambless LE, Bond G. Carotid artery intimal-medial wall thickening and plasma homocyst(e)ine in asymptomatic adults. The Atherosclerosis Risk in Communities Study. *Circulation* 1993;87:1107-1113.

165. Bots ML, Launer LJ, Lindemans J, Hofman A, Grobbee DE. Homocysteine, atherosclerosis and prevalent cardiovascular disease in the elderly: The Rotterdam Study. *J Intern Med* 1997;242:339-347.

166. Markus H, Kapozsta Z, Ditrich R, et al. Increased common carotid intima-media thickness in UK African Caribbeans and its relation to chronic inflammation and vascular candidate gene polymorphisms. *Stroke* 2001;32:2465-2471.

167. Durga J, Bots ML, Schouten EG, Grobbee DE, Kok FJ, Verhoef P. Homocysteine not associated with intima-media thickness. *J Inherit Metab Dis* 2003;26(Suppl.1):25.

168. Vermeer SE, van Dijk EJ, Koudstaal PJ, et al. Homocysteine, silent brain infarcts, and white matter lesions: The Rotterdam Scan Study. *Ann Neurol* 2002;51:285-289.

169. Inamoto N, Katsuya T, Kokubo Y, et al. Association of methylenetetrahydrofolate reductase gene polymorphism with carotid atherosclerosis depending on smoking status in a Japanese general population. *Stroke* 2003;34:1628-1633.

170. Passaro A, Vanini A, Calzoni F, et al. Plasma homocysteine, methylenetetrahydrofolate reductase mutation and carotid damage in elderly healthy women. *Atherosclerosis* 2001;157:175-180.

171. Willinek WA, Ludwig M, Lennarz M, Höller T, Stumpe KO. High-normal serum homocysteine concentrations are associated with an increased risk of early atherosclerotic carotid artery wall lesions in healthy subjects. *J Hypertens* 2000;18:425-430.

172. Majors AK, Pyeritz RE. A deficiency of cysteine impairs fibrillin-1 deposition: implications for the pathogenesis of cystathionine β-synthase deficiency. *Mol Genet Metab* 2000;70:252-260.

173. Ducloux D, Motte G, Challier B, Gibey R, Chalopin J-M. Serum total homocysteine and cardiovascular disease occurrence in chronic, stable renal transplant recipients: a prospective study. *J Am Soc Nephrol* 2000;11:134-137.

174. Han H, Dwyer JT, Selhub J, et al. Serum cystatin C is an independent predictor of total homocysteine levels in stable Korean renal transplant recipients with normal serum creatinine. *J Ren Nutr* 2001;11:149-154.

175. Lasseur C, Parrot F, Delmas Y, et al. Impact of high-flux/high-efficiency dialysis on folate and homocysteine metabolism. *J Nephrol* 2001;14:32-35.

176. Jennette JC, Goldman ID. Inhibition of the membrane transport of folates by anions retained in uremia. *J Lab Clin Med* 1975;86:834-843.

177. Livant EJ, Tamura T, Johnston KE, et al. Plasma folate conjugase activities and folate concentrations in patients receiving hemodialysis. *J Nutr Biochem* 1994;5:504-508.

178. Bostom AG, Shemin D, Lapane KL, et al. Hyperhomocysteinemia and traditional cardiovascular disease risk factors in end-stage renal disease patients on dialysis: a case-control study. *Atherosclerosis* 1995;114:93-103.

179. Bostom AG, Shemin D, Gohh RY, et al. Treatment of hyperhomocysteinemia in hemodialysis patients and renal transplant recipients. *Kidney Int* 2001;59 (Suppl 78):S246-S252.

180. Lim PS, Hung WR, Wei YH. Polymorphism in methylenetetrahydrofolate reductase gene: Its impact on plasma homocysteine levels and carotid atherosclerosis in ESRD patients receiving hemodialysis. *Nephron* 2001;87:249-256.

181. Haraki T, Takegoshi T, Kitoh C, et al. Hyperhomocysteinemia, diabetes mellitus, and carotid atherosclerosis independently increase atherosclerotic vascular disease outcome in Japanese patients with end-stage renal disease. *Clin Nephrol* 2001;56:132-139.

182. Oh J, Wunsch R, Turzer M, et al. Advanced coronary and carotid arteriopathy in young adults with childhood-onset chronic renal failure. *Circulation* 2002;106:100-105.

183. Brzósko S, Lebkowska U, Malyszko J, Hryszko T, Pawlak K, Mysliwiec M. Correlation between carotid intima-media thickness and hematocrit and hemoglobin values in renal transplant recipients. *Clin Transplant* 2001;15:349-353.

184. Zoungas S, Ristevski S, Lightfoot P, et al. Proceedings of the High Blood Pressure Research Council of Australia - Carotid artery intima-medial thickness is increased in chronic renal failure. *Clin Exp Pharmacol Physiol* 2000;27:639-641.

185. Kennedy R, Case C, Fathi R, Johnson D, Isbel N, Marwick TH. Does renal failure cause an atherosclerotic milieu in patients with end-stage renal disease? *Am J Med* 2001;110:198-204.

186. Libetta C, Villa G, Pirrelli S, et al. Homocysteine plasma levels correlate with intimal carotid artery thickness in haemodialysis patients. *Nephrol Dial Transplant* 2001;16:2444-2445.

187. Maeda N, Sawayama Y, Tatsukawa M, et al. Carotid artery lesions and atherosclerotic risk factors in Japanese hemodialysis patients. *Atherosclerosis* 2003;169:183-192.

188. Schwarz U, Buzello M, Ritz E, et al. Morphology of coronary atherosclerotic lesions in patients with end-stage renal failure. *Nephrol Dial Transplant* 2000;15:218-223.

189. Raal FJ, Areias AJ, Waisberg R, von Arb M. Susceptibility of low density lipo-protein to oxidation in familial hypercholesterolaemia. *Atherosclerosis* 1995;115:9-15.

190. Paiker JE, Raal FJ, von Arb M. Auto-antibodies against oxidized LDL as a marker of coronary artery disease in patients with familial hypercholesterolaemia. *Ann Clin Biochem* 2000;37:174-178.

191. Zhou J, Moller J, Danielsen CC, et al. Dietary supplementation with methionine and homocysteine promotes early atherosclerosis but not plaque rupture in ApoE-deficient mice. *Arterioscler Thromb Vasc Biol* 2001;21:1470-1476.

192. Audelin MC, Genest J. Homocysteine and cardiovascular disease in diabetes mellitus. *Atherosclerosis* 2001;159:497-511.

193. Fonseca VA, Mudaliar S, Schmidt B, Fink LM, Kern PA, Henry RR. Plasma homocysteine concentrations are regulated by acute hyperinsulinemia in nondiabetic but not type 2 diabetic subjects. *Metabolism* 1998;47:686-689.

194. Hofmann MA, Kohl B, Zumbach MS, et al. Hyperhomocyst(e)inemia and endothelial dysfunction in IDDM. *Diabetes Care* 1998;21:841-848.

195. Wollesen F, Brattström L, Refsum H, Ueland PM, Berglund L, Berne C. Plasma total homocysteine and cysteine in relation to glomerular filtration rate in diabetes mellitus. *Kidney Int* 1999;55:1028-1035.

196. House JD, Jacobs RL, Stead LM, Brosnan ME, Brosnan JT. Regulation of homocysteine metabolism. *Adv Enzyme Regul* 1999;39:69-91.

197. Petri M. Treatment of systemic lupus erythematosus: an update. *Am Fam Physician* 1998;57:2753-2760.

198. Petri M, Roubenoff R, Dallal GE, Nadeau MR, Selhub J, Rosenberg IH. Plasma homocysteine as a risk factor for atherothrombotic events in systemic lupus erythematosus. *Lancet* 1996;348:1120-1124.

199. Roman MJ, Salmon JE, Sobel R, et al. Prevalence and relation to risk factors of carotid atherosclerosis and left ventricular hypertrophy in systemic lupus erythematosus and antiphospholipid antibody syndrome. *Am J Cardiol* 2001;87:663-666.

200. Miller JW, Shukitt-Hale B, Villalobos-Molina R, Nadeau MR, Selhub J, Joseph JA. Effect of L-Dopa and the catechol-O-methyltransferase inhibitor Ro 41-0960 on sulfur amino acid metabolites in rats. *Clin Neuropharmacol* 1997;20:55-66.

201. Blandini F, Fancellu R, Martignoni E, et al. Plasma homocysteine and L-DOPA metabolism in patients with Parkinson disease. *Clin Chem* 2001;47:1102-1104.

202. Frosst P, Blom HJ, Milos R, et al. A candidate genetic risk factor for vascular disease: a common mutation in methylenetetrahydrofolate reductase. *Nat Genet* 1995;10:111-113.

203. Guenther BD, Sheppard CA, Tran P, Rozen R, Matthews RG, Ludwig ML. The structure and properties of methylenetetrahydrofolate reductase from *Escherichia coli* suggest how folate ameliorates human hyperhomocysteinemia. *Nat Struct Biol* 1999;6:359-365.

204. Fohr IP, Prinz-Langenohl R., Brönstrup A, et al. 5,10-methylenetetrahydrofolate reductase genotype determines the plasma homocysteine-lowering effect of supplementation with 5-methyltetrahydrofolate or folic acid in healthy young women. *Am J Clin Nutr* 2002;75:275-282.

205. Matthews RG, Kaufman S. Characterization of the dihydropterin reductase activity of pig liver methylenetetrahydrofolate reductase. *J Biol Chem* 1980;255:6014-6017.

206. Kaufman S. Some metabolic relationships between biopterin and folate: implications for the "methyl trap hypothesis". *Neurochem Res* 1991;16:1031-1036.

207. Bagley PJ, Selhub J. A common mutation in the methylenetetrahydrofolate reductase gene is associated with an accumulation of formylated tetrahydrofolates in red blood cells. *Proc Natl Acad Sci U S A* 1998;95:13217-13220.

208. Verhaar MC, Stroes E, Rabelink TJ. Folates and cardiovascular disease. *Arterioscler Thromb Vasc Biol* 2002;22:6-13.

209. Arai K, Yamasaki Y, Kajimoto Y, et al. Association of methylenetetrahydrofolate reductase gene polymorphism with carotid arterial wall thickening and myocardial infarction risk in NIDDM. *Diabetes* 1997;46:2102-2104.

210. Ravera M, Viazzi F, Berruti V, et al. 5,10-Methylenetetrahydrofolate reductase polymorphism and early organ damage in primary hypertension. *Am J Hypertens* 2001;14:371-376.

211. Pallaud C, Sass C, Zannad F, Siest G, Visvikis S. APOC3, CETP, fibrinogen, and MTHFR are genetic determinants of carotid intima-media thickness in healthy men (the Stanislas cohort). *Clin Genet* 2001;59:316-324.

212. Kawamoto R, Kohara K, Tabara Y, et al. An association of 5,10-methylenetetrahydrofolate reductase (*MTHFR*) gene polymorphism and common carotid atherosclerosis. *J Hum Genet* 2001;46:506-510.

213. Zuliani G, Volpato S, Mecocci P, Cherubini A. The A677V MTHFR allele is not associated with carotid atherosclerosis in octogenarians. *Stroke* 2000;31:990-991.

214. Chern C-L, Huang R-FS, Chen Y-H, Cheng J-T, Liu T-Z. Folate deficiency-induced oxidative stress and apoptosis are mediated via homocysteine-dependent overproduction of hydrogen peroxide and enhanced activation of NF-κB in human Hep G2 cells. *Biomed Pharmacother* 2001;55:434-442.

215. Hofmann MA, Lalla E, Lu Y, et al. Hyperhomocysteinemia enhances vascular inflammation and accelerates atherosclerosis in a murine model. *J Clin Invest* 2001;107:675-683.

216. Zeitlin A, Frishman WH, Chang CJ. The association of vitamin B_{12} and folate blood levels with mortality and cardiovascular morbidity incidence in the old old: the Bronx aging study. *Am J Ther* 1997;4:275-281.

217. Spence JD. Ultrasound measurement of carotid plaque as a surrogate outcome for coronary artery disease. *Am J Cardiol* 2002;89:10B-16B.

218. del Sol AI, Bots ML, Grobbee DE, Hofman A, Witteman JCM. Carotid intima-media thickness at different sites: relation to incident myocardial infarction - The Rotterdam Study. *Eur Heart J* 2002;23:934-940.

219. Morita H, Kurihara H, Yoshida S, et al. Diet-induced hyperhomocysteinemia exacerbates neointima formation in rat carotid arteries after balloon injury. *Circulation* 2001;103:133-139.

220. Lentz SR, Piegors DJ, Malinow MR, Heistad DD. Supplementation of atherogenic diet with B vitamins does not prevent atherosclerosis or vascular dysfunction in monkeys. *Circulation* 2001;103:1006-1011.

221. Vermeulen EGJ, Niessen HWM, Bogels M, Stehouwer CDA, Rauwerda JA, van Hinsbergh VWM. Decreased smooth muscle cell/extracellular matrix ratio of media of femoral artery in patients with atherosclerosis and hyperhomocysteinemia. *Arterioscler Thromb Vasc Biol* 2001;21:573-577.

222. Jacobsen DW. Hyperhomocysteinemia and oxidative stress: time for a reality check? *Arterioscler Thromb Vasc Biol* 2000;20:1182-1184.

223. Welch GN, Upchurch GR, Farivar RS, et al. Homocysteine-induced nitric oxide production in vascular smooth-muscle cells by NF-κB-dependent transcriptional activation of *Nos2*. *Proc Assoc Am Physicians* 1998;110:22-31.

224. Duan J, Murohara T, Ikeda H, et al. Hyperhomocysteinemia impairs angiogenesis in response to hindlimb ischemia. *Arterioscler Thromb Vasc Biol* 2000;20:2579-2585.

225. Bagi Z, Ungvari Z, Szollár L, Koller A. Flow-induced constriction in arterioles of hyperhomocysteinemic rats is due to impaired nitric oxide and enhanced thromboxane A_2 mediation. *Arterioscler Thromb Vasc Biol* 2001;21:233-237.

226. Tsai JC, Perrella MA, Yoshizumi M, et al. Promotion of vascular smooth muscle cell growth by homocysteine: a link to atherosclerosis. *Proc Natl Acad Sci U S A* 1994;91:6369-6373.

227. Toborek M, Kopieczna-Grzebieniak E, Drózdz M, Wieczorek M. Increased lipid peroxidation as a mechanism of methionine-induced atherosclerosis in rabbits. *Atherosclerosis* 1995;115:217-224.

228. Chen C, Surowiec SM, Morsy AH, Ma M. Intraperitoneal infusion of homocysteine increases intimal hyperplasia in balloon-injured rat carotid arteries. *Atherosclerosis* 2002;160:103-114.

229. Charpiot P, Bescond A, Augier T, et al. Hyperhomocysteinemia induces elastolysis in minipig arteries: structural consequences, arterial site specificity and effect of captopril-hydrochlorothiazide. *Matrix Biol* 1998;17:559-574.

230. Durand P, Prost M, Blache D. Pro-thrombotic effects of a folic acid deficient diet in rat platelets and macrophages related to elevated homocysteine and decreased n-3 polyunsaturated fatty acids. *Atherosclerosis* 1996;121:231-243.

231. Jakubowski H, Zhang L, Bardeguez A, Aviv A. Homocysteine thiolactone and protein homocysteinylation in human endothelial cells: implications for atherosclerosis. *Circ Res* 2000;87:45-51.

232. Böger RH, Bode-Böger SM, Sydow K, Heistad DD, Lentz SR. Plasma concentration of asymmetric dimethylarginine, an endogenous inhibitor of nitric oxide synthase, is elevated in monkeys with hyperhomocyst(e)inemia or hypercholesterolemia. *Arterioscler Thromb Vasc Biol* 2000;20:1557-1564.

233. Ambrosi P, Rolland PH, Bodard H, et al. Effects of folate supplementation in hyperhomocysteinemic pigs. *J Am Coll Cardiol* 1999;34:274-279.

234. Smith TP, Cruz CP, Brown AT, Eidt JF, Moursi MM. Folate supplementation inhibits intimal hyperplasia induced by a high-homocysteine diet in a rat carotid endarterectomy model. *J Vasc Surg* 2001;34:474-481.

235. Clarke R, Armitage J. Vitamin supplements and cardiovascular risk: review of the randomized trials of homocysteine-lowering vitamin supplements. *Semin Thromb Hemost* 2000;26:341-348.

236. Clarke R, Collins R. Can dietary supplements with folic acid or vitamin B_6 reduce cardiovascular risk? Design of clinical trials to test the homocysteine hypothesis of vascular disease. *J Cardiovasc Risk* 1998;5:249-255.

237. Robinson K, Arheart K, Refsum H, et al. Low circulating folate and vitamin B_6 concentrations: risk factors for stroke, peripheral vascular disease, and coronary artery disease. *Circulation* 1998;97:437-443.

238. Durga J, Verhoef P, Bots ML, Schouten EG. Homocysteine and carotid intima-media thickness: a critical appraisal of the evidence. *Atherosclerosis* 2004;176:1-19.

239. Greenland P, Abrams J, Aurigemma GP, et al. Prevention Conference V: Beyond secondary prevention: identifying the high-risk patient for primary prevention: noninvasive tests of atherosclerotic burden: Writing Group III. *Circulation* 2000;101:E16-E22.

240. Nichols, W. M. *McDonald's Blood Flow in Arteries: Theoretical, Experimental and Clinical Principles.* Nichols, W. M. and O'Rourke, M. F. 4th edition. 1998. London, UK: Edward Arnold.

241. van Guldener C, Lambert J, Janssen MJFM, Donker AJM, Stehouwer CDA. Endothelium-dependent vasodilatation and distensibility of large arteries in chronic haemodialysis patients. *Nephrol Dial Transplant* 1997;12(Suppl 2):14-18.

242. Ubbink JB, Hayward-Vermaak WJ, Bissbort S. Rapid high-performance liquid chromatographic assay for total homocysteine levels in human serum. *J Chromatogr* 1991;565:441-446.

243. Schuit AJ, Schouten EG, Westerterp KR, Saris WH. Validity of the Physical Acitivity Scale for the Elderly (PASE): According to energy expenditure assessed by the doubly labeled water method. *J Clin Epidemiol* 1997;50:541-546.

244. Voorlichtingsbureau voor de Voeding. *Zo eet Nederland. Resultaten van de voedselconsumptiepeiling 1992.* 1993.

245. Institute of Medicine. *Dietary reference intakes for thiamin, riboflavin, niacin, vitamin B_6, folate, vitamin B_{12}, panthothenic acid, biotin, and choline.* 150-305. 1-1-1998. National Academy Press. Recommended Dietary Allowances.

246. Symons JD, Mullick AE, Ensunsa JL, Ma AA, Rutledge JC. Hyperhomocysteinemia evoked by folate depletion: effects on coronary and carotid arterial function. *Arterioscler Thromb Vasc Biol* 2002;22:772-780.

247. Rolland PH, Friggi A, Barlatier A, et al. Hyperhomocysteinemia-induced vascular damage in the minipig. Captopril-hydrochlorothiazide combination prevents elastic alterations. *Circulation* 1995;91:1161-1174.

248. Baumbach GL, Sigmund CD, Bottiglieri T, Lentz SR. Structure of cerebral arterioles in cystathionine β-synthase-deficient mice. *Circ Res* 2002;91:931-937.

249. Chambless LE, Folsom AR, Davis V, et al. Risk factors for progression of common carotid atherosclerosis: the Atherosclerosis Risk in Communities Study, 1987-1998. *Am J Epidemiol* 2002;155:38-47.

250. Bots ML, Hoes AW, Koudstaal PJ, Hofman A, Grobbee DE. Common carotid intima-media thickness and risk of stroke and myocardial infarction: the Rotterdam Study. *Circulation* 1997;96:1432-1437.

251. Herbert V. Experimental nutritional folate deficiency in man. *Trans Assoc Am Physicians* 1962;75:307-320.

252. Botez MI, Botez T, Maag U. The Wechsler subtests in mild organic brain damage associated with folate deficiency. *Psychol Med* 1984;14:431-437.

253. Pasquier F, Lebert F, Petit H, Zittoun J, Marquet J. Methylenetetrahydrofolate reductase deficiency revealed by a neuropathy in a psychotic adult. *J Neurol Neurosurg Psychiatry* 1994;57:765-766.

254. Reynolds EH. Effects of folic acid on the mental state and fit-frequency of drug-treated epileptic patients. *Lancet* 1967;1:1086-1088.

255. Botez MI, Fontaine F, Botez T, Bachevalier J. Folate-responsive neurological and mental disorders: report of 16 cases. Neuropsychological correlates of computerized transaxial tomography and radionuclide cisternography in folic acid deficiencies. *Eur Neurol* 1977;16:230-246.

256. Enk C, Hougaard K, Hippe E. Reversible dementia and neuropathy associated with folate deficiency 16 years after partial gastrectomy. *Scand J Haematol* 1980;25:63-66.

257. Freeman JM, Finkelstein JD, Mudd SH. Folate-responsive homocystinuria and "schizophrenia." A defect in methylation due to deficient 5,10-methylene-tetrahydrofolate reductase activity. *N Engl J Med* 1975;292:491-496.

258. Manzoor M, Runcie J. Folate-responsive neuropathy: report of 10 cases. *Br Med J* 1976;1:1176-1178.

259. Strachan RW, Henderson JG. Dementia and folate deficiency. *Q J Med* 1967;36:189-204.

260. Brookes PS, Baggott JE. Oxidation of 10-formyltetrahydrofolate to 10-formyldihydrofolate by complex IV of rat mitochondria. *Biochemistry* 2002;41:5633-5636.

261. Emerit J, Edeas M, Bricaire F. Neurodegenerative diseases and oxidative stress. *Biomed Pharmacother* 2004;58:39-46.

262. Riggs KM, Spiro A, Tucker K, Rush D. Relations of vitamin B-12, vitamin B-6, folate, and homocysteine to cognitive performance in the Normative Aging Study. *Am J Clin Nutr* 1996;63:306-314.

263. McCaddon A, Hudson P, Davies G, Hughes A, Williams JH, Wilkinson C. Homocysteine and cognitive decline in healthy elderly. *Dement Geriatr Cogn Disord* 2001;12:309-313.

264. Teunissen CE, Lütjohann D, von Bergmann K, et al. Combination of serum markers related to several mechanisms in Alzheimer's disease. *Neurobiol Aging* 2003;24:893-902.

265. Seshadri S, Beiser A, Selhub J, et al. Plasma homocysteine as a risk factor for dementia and Alzheimer's disease. *N Engl J Med* 2002;346:476-483.

266. Breteler MMB, Claus JJ, Grobbee DE, Hofman A. Cardiovascular disease and distribution of cognitive function in elderly people: the Rotterdam Study. *Br Med J* 1994;308:1604-1608.

267. Hofman A, Ott A, Breteler MM, et al. Atherosclerosis, apolipoprotein E, and prevalence of dementia and Alzheimer's disease in the Rotterdam Study. *Lancet* 1997;349:151-154.

268. van Exel E, Gussekloo J, Houx P, et al. Atherosclerosis and cognitive impairment are linked in the elderly. The Leiden 85-plus Study. *Atherosclerosis* 2002;165:353-359.

269. Auperin A, Berr C, Bonithon KC, et al. Ultrasonographic assessment of carotid wall characteristics and cognitive functions in a community sample of 59- to 71-year-olds. The EVA Study Group. *Stroke* 1996;27:1290-1295.

270. Krupenko SA, Oleinik NV. 10-formyltetrahydrofolate dehydrogenase, one of the major folate enzymes, is down-regulated in tumor tissues and possesses suppressor effects on cancer cells. *Cell Growth Differ* 2002;13:227-236.

271. Oleinik NV, Krupenko SA. Ectopic expression of 10-formyltetrahydrofolate dehydrogenase in A549 cells induces G_1 cell cycle arrest and apoptosis. *Mol Cancer Res* 2003;1:577-588.

272. Barbaux S, Plomin R, Whitehead AS. Polymorphisms of genes controlling homocysteine/folate metabolism and cognitive function. *Neuroreport* 2000;11:1133-1136.

273. Visscher PM, Tynan M, Whiteman MC, et al. Lack of association between polymorphisms in angiotensin-converting-enzyme and methylenetetrahydrofolate reductase genes and normal cognitive ageing in humans. *Neurosci Lett* 2003;347:175-178.

274. Methods II: Measurements. In: Jolles J, Houx PJ, van Boxtel MPJ, Ponds RWHM, eds. *Maastricht Aging Study: Determinants of cognitive aging.* Maastricht: Neuropsych Publishers, 1995:25-38.

275. Folstein MF, Folstein SE, McHugh PR. "Mini-mental state". A practical method for grading the cognitive state of patients for the clinician. *J Psychiatr Res* 1975;12:189-198.

276. Morris MS, Jacques PF, Rosenberg IH, Selhub J. Hyperhomocysteinemia associated with poor recall in the third National Health and Nutrition Examination Survey. *Am J Clin Nutr* 2001;73:927-933.

277. Duthie SJ, Whalley LJ, Collins AR, Leaper S, Berger K, Deary IJ. Homocysteine, B vitamin status, and cognitive function in the elderly. *Am J Clin Nutr* 2002;75:908-913.

278. La Rue A, Koehler KM, Wayne SJ, Chiulli SJ, Haaland KY, Garry PJ. Nutritional status and cognitive functioning in a normally aging sample: a 6-y reassessment. *Am J Clin Nutr* 1997;65:20-29.

279. Tobin MD, Minelli C, Burton PR, Thompson JR. Commentary: development of Mendelian randomization: from hypothesis test to 'Mendelian deconfounding'. *Int J Epidemiol* 2004;33:26-29.

280. Osmond H, Smythies JR. Schizophrenia: new approaches. *J Ment Sci* 1952;98:309-315.

281. Chen Z, Karaplis AC, Ackerman SL, et al. Mice deficient in methylenetetrahydrofolate reductase exhibit hyperhomocysteinemia and decreased

methylation capacity, with neuropathology and aortic lipid deposition. *Hum Mol Genet* 2001;10:433-443.

282. Hyland K, Smith I, Bottiglieri T, et al. Demyelination and decreased S-adenosylmethionine in 5,10-methylenetetrahydrofolate reductase deficiency. *Neurology* 1988;38:459-462.

283. Fontanari D, Di-Palma C, Giorgetti G, Violante F, Voltolina M. Effects of S-adenosyl-L-methionine on cognitive and vigilance functions in the elderly. *Curr Ther Res Clin Exp* 1994;55:682-689.

284. Marcus EL, Berry EM. Refusal to eat in the elderly. *Nutr Rev* 1998;56:163-171.

285. Rosen S, Olin P. Hearing loss and coronary heart disease. *Bull N Y Acad Med* 1965;41:1052-1068.

286. Gates GA, Cooper JC. Incidence of hearing decline in the elderly. *Acta Oto-Laryngol* 1991;111:240-248.

287. Seidman MD, Ahmad N, Bai U. Molecular mechanisms of age-related hearing loss. *Ageing Res Rev* 2002;1:331-343.

288. Cortopassi G, Hutchin T. A molecular and cellular hypothesis for aminoglycoside-induced deafness. *Hear Res* 1994;78:27-30.

289. Johnsson L-G, Hawkins JE Jr. Vascular changes in the human inner ear associated with aging. *Ann Otol Rhinol Laryngol* 1972;81:364-376.

290. Makishima K. Arteriolar sclerosis as a cause of presbycusis. *Otolaryngology* 1978;86:ORL322-ORL326.

291. Podoshin L, Fradis M, Pillar T, Zisman D. Senso-neural hearing loss as an expression of atherosclerosis in young people. *Eye Ear Nose Throat Mon* 1975;54:18-23.

292. Rubinstein M, Hildesheimer M, Zohar S, Chilarovitz T. Chronic cardiovascular pathology and hearing loss in the aged. *Gerontology* 1977;23:4-9.

293. Parving A, Hein HO, Suadicani P, Ostri B, Gyntelberg F. Epidemiology of hearing disorders. Some factors affecting hearing. The Copenhagen Male Study. *Scand Audiol* 1993;22:101-107.

294. Susmano A, Rosenbush SW. Hearing loss and ischemic heart disease. *Am J Otol* 1988;9:403-408.

295. Gates GA, Cobb JL, D'Agostino RB, Wolf PA. The relation of hearing in the elderly to the presence of cardiovascular disease and cardiovascular risk factors. *Arch Otolaryngol Head Neck Surg* 1993;119:156-161.

296. Bild DE, Fitzpatrick A, Fried LP, et al. Age-related trends in cardiovascular morbidity and physical functioning in the elderly: the Cardiovascular Health Study. *J Am Geriatr Soc* 1993;41:1047-1056.

297. Hariri MA, Lakshmi MV, Larner S, Connolly MJ. Auditory problems in elderly patients with stroke. *Age Ageing* 1994;23:312-316.

298. Brant LJ, Gordon-Salant S, Pearson JD, et al. Risk factors related to age-associated hearing loss in the speech frequencies. *J Am Acad Audiol* 1996;7:152-160.

299. Fuortes LJ, Tang S, Pomrehn P, Anderson C. Prospective evaluation of associations between hearing sensitivity and selected cardiovascular risk factors. *Am J Ind Med* 1995;28:275-280.

300. Maggi S, Minicuci N, Martini A, et al. Prevalence rates of hearing impairment and comorbid conditions in older people: the Veneto Study. *J Am Geriatr Soc* 1998;46:1069-1074.

301. Drettner B, Hedstrand H, Klockhoff I, Svedberg A. Cardiovascular risk factors and hearing loss. A study of 1,000 fifty-year-old men. *Acta Oto-Laryngol* 1975;79:366-371.

302. Chen YL, Ding YP. Relationship between hypertension and hearing disorders in the elderly. *East Afr Med J* 1999;76:344-347.

303. Cruickshanks KJ, Klein R, Klein BEK, Wiley TL, Nondahl DM, Tweed TS. Cigarette smoking and hearing loss: The epidemiology of hearing loss study. *J Am Med Assoc* 1998;279:1715-1719.

304. Tawakol A, Forgione MA, Stuehlinger M, et al. Homocysteine impairs coronary microvascular dilator function in humans. *J Am Coll Cardiol* 2002;40:1051-1058.

305. Lipton SA, Kim WK, Choi YB, et al. Neurotoxicity associated with dual actions of homocysteine at the N-methyl-D-aspartate receptor. *Proc Natl Acad Sci U S A* 1997;94:5923-5928.

306. Puel JL, Ladrech S, Chabert R, Pujol R, Eybalin M. Electrophysiological evidence for the presence of NMDA receptors in the guinea pig cochlea. *Hear Res* 1991;51:255-264.

307. Jacques PF, Bostom AG, Williams RR, et al. Relation between folate status, a common mutation in methylenetetrahydrofolate reductase, and plasma homocysteine concentrations. *Circulation* 1996;93:7-9.

308. Verhaar MC, Wever RMF, Kastelein JJP, van Dam T, Koomans HA, Rabelink TJ. 5-methyltetrahydrofolate, the active form of folic acid, restores endothelial function in familial hypercholesterolemia. *Circulation* 1998;97:237-241.

309. Covell WP. Pathologic changes in the peripheral auditory mechanism due to avitaminoses (A, B complex, C, D and E). *Laryngoscope* 1940;2:632-647.

310. Hughson, W and Westlake, H. *Manual for program outline for rehabilitation of aural casualities both military and civilian.* 1944. Rochester, New York, U.S.A., American Academy of Ophtalmologists and Otologists.

311. van Popele NM, Grobbee DE, Bots ML, et al. Association between arterial stiffness and atherosclerosis - The Rotterdam study. *Stroke* 2001;32:454-460.

312. Cruickshanks KJ, Tweed TS, Wiley TL, et al. The 5-year incidence and progression of hearing loss: the epidemiology of hearing loss study. *Arch Otolaryngol Head Neck Surg* 2003;129:1041-1046.

313. Ross R. Atherosclerosis--an inflammatory disease. *N Engl J Med* 1999;340:115-126.

314. Libby P. Inflammation in atherosclerosis. *Nature* 2002;420:868-874.

315. Zhang R, Ma J, Xia M, Zhu H, Ling W. Mild hyperhomocysteinemia induced by feeding rats diets rich in methionine or deficient in folate promotes early atherosclerotic inflammatory processes. *J Nutr* 2004;134:825-830.

316. Wang G, Woo CWH, Sung FL, Siow YL, O K. Increased monocyte adhesion to aortic endothelium in rats with hyperhomocysteinemia: role of chemokine and adhesion molecules. *Arterioscler Thromb Vasc Biol* 2002;22:1777-1783.

317. Lee H, Kim HJ, Kim J, Chang N. Effects of dietary folic acid supplementation on cerebrovascular endothelial dysfunction in rats with induced hyperhomocysteinemia. *Brain Res* 2004;996:139-147.

318. Powers RW, Majors AK, Cerula SL, Huber HA, Schmidt BP, Roberts JM. Changes in markers of vascular injury in response to transient hyperhomocysteinemia. *Metabolism* 2003;52:501-507.

319. Holven KB, Scholz H, Halvorsen B, Aukrust P, Ose L, Nenseter MS. Hyperhomocysteinemic subjects have enhanced expression of lectin-like oxidized LDL receptor-1 in mononuclear cells. *J Nutr* 2003;133:3588-3591.

320. Leeuwenberg JF, Smeets EF, Neefjes JJ, et al. E-selectin and intercellular adhesion molecule-1 are released by activated human endothelial cells in vitro. *Immunology* 1992;77:543-549.

321. Holvoet P, Donck J, Landeloos M, et al. Correlation between oxidized low density lipoproteins and von Willebrand factor in chronic renal failure. *Thromb Haemost* 1996;76:663-669.

322. van Tits LJH, de Waart F, Hak Lemmers HLM, et al. Effects of α-tocopherol on superoxide production and plasma intercellular adhesion molecule-1 and antibodies to oxidized LDL in chronic smokers. *Free Radic Biol Med* 2001;30:1122-1129.

323. Chao C-L, Kuo T-L, Lee Y-T. Effects of methionine-induced hyperhomocysteinemia on endothelium-dependent vasodilation and oxidative status in healthy adults. *Circulation* 2000;101:485-490.

324. Steinberg D, Witztum JL. Is the oxidative modification hypothesis relevant to human atherosclerosis? Do the antioxidant trials conducted to date refute the hypothesis? *Circulation* 2002;105:2107-2111.

325. Hackam DG, Anand SS. Emerging risk factors for atherosclerotic vascular disease: a critical review of the evidence. *J Am Med Assoc* 2003;290:932-940.

326. Ridker PM, Hennekens CH, Roitman-Johnson B, Stampfer MJ, Allen J. Plasma concentration of soluble intercellular adhesion molecule 1 and risks of future myocardial infarction in apparently healthy men. *Lancet* 1998;351:88-92.

327. Holvoet P, Harris TB, Tracy RP, et al. Association of high coronary heart disease risk status with circulating oxidized LDL in the well-functioning elderly: findings from the Health, Aging, and Body Composition study. *Arterioscler Thromb Vasc Biol* 2003;23:1444-1448.

328. Salonen JT, Ylä-Herttuala S, Yamamoto R, et al. Autoantibody against oxidised LDL and progression of carotid atherosclerosis. *Lancet* 1992;339:883-887.

329. Puurunen M, Manttari M, Manninen V, et al. Antibody against oxidized low-density lipoprotein predicting myocardial infarction. *Arch Intern Med* 1994;154:2605-2609.

330. Rossi GP, Cesari M, De Toni R, et al. Antibodies to oxidized low-density lipoproteins and angiographically assessed coronary artery disease in white patients. *Circulation* 2003;108:2467-2472.

331. Lopes-Virella MF, Binzafar N, Rackley S, Takei A, La Via M, Virella G. The uptake of LDL-IC by human macrophages: predominant involvement of the FcγRI receptor. *Atherosclerosis* 1997;135:161-170.

332. Hörkkö S, Binder CJ, Shaw PX, et al. Immunological responses to oxidized LDL. *Free Radic Biol Med* 2000;28:1771-1779.

333. Shaw PX, Horkko S, Tsimikas S, et al. Human-derived anti-oxidized LDL autoantibody blocks uptake of oxidized LDL by macrophages and localizes to atherosclerotic lesions in vivo. *Arterioscler Thromb Vasc Biol* 2001;21:1333-1339.

334. Miller YI, Chang M-K, Binder CJ, Shaw PX, Witztum JL. Oxidized low density lipoprotein and innate immune receptors. *Curr Opin Lipidol* 2003;14:437-445.

335. Chiarello PG, Vannucchi MTI, Moysés Neto M, Vannucchi H. Hyperhomocysteinemia and oxidative stress in hemodialysis: effects of supplementation with folic acid. *Int J Vitam Nutr Res* 2003;73:431-438.

336. Bayés B, Pastor MC, Bonal J, Juncà J, Romero R. Homocysteine and lipid peroxidation in haemodialysis: role of folinic acid and vitamin E. *Nephrol Dial Transplant* 2001;16:2172-2175.

337. Apeland T, Mansoor MA, Seljeflot I, Brønstad I, Gøransson L, Strandjord RE. Homocysteine, malondialdehyde and endothelial markers in dialysis patients during low-dose folinic acid therapy. *J Intern Med* 2002;252:456-464.

338. Church TS, Earnest CP, Wood KA, Kampert JB. Reduction of C-reactive protein levels through use of a multivitamin. *Am J Med* 2003;115:702-707.

339. Jang Y, Lee JH, Kim OY, Park HY, Lee SY. Consumption of whole grain and legume powder reduces insulin demand, lipid peroxidation, and plasma homocysteine concentrations in patients with coronary artery disease: randomized controlled clinical trial. *Arterioscler Thromb Vasc Biol* 2001;21:2065-2071.

340. Carson NAJ, Neill DW. Metabolic abnormalities detected in a survey of mentally backward individuals in Northern Ireland. *Arch Dis Childhood* 1962;37:505-513.

341. Gerritsen T, Vaughn JG, Waisman HA. Identification of homocysteine in urine. *Biochem Biophys Res Commun* 1962;9:493-496.

342. Mudd SH, Finkelstein JD, Irreverre F, Laster L. Homocystinuria: an enzyme defect. *Science* 1964;143:1443-1445.

343. Thambyrajah J, Townend JN. Homocysteine and atherothrombosis--mechanisms for injury. *Eur Heart J* 2000;21:967-974.

344. Bennett-Richards K, Kattenhorn M, Donald A, et al. Does oral folic acid lower total homocysteine levels and improve endothelial function in children with chronic renal failure? *Circulation* 2002;105:1810-1815.

345. Alul RH, Wood M, Longo J, et al. Vitamin C protects low-density lipoprotein from homocysteine-mediated oxidation. *Free Radic Biol Med* 2003;34:881-891.

346. Kanani PM, Sinkey CA, Browning RL, Allaman M, Knapp HR, Haynes WG. Role of oxidant stress in endothelial dysfunction produced by experimental hyperhomocyst(e)inemia in humans. *Circulation* 1999;100:1161-1168.

347. Nakano E, Williamson MP, Williams NH, Powers HJ. Copper-mediated LDL oxidation by homocysteine and related compounds depends largely on copper ligation. *Biochim Biophys Acta* 2004;1688:33-42.

348. Earnest CP, Wood KA, Church TS. Complex multivitamin supplementation improves homocysteine and resistance to LDL-C oxidation. *J Am Coll Nutr* 2003;22:400-407.

349. Goodwin JS, Goodwin JM, Garry PJ. Association between nutritional status and cognitive functioning in a healthy elderly population. *J Am Med Assoc* 1983;249:2917-2921.

350. Ho PI, Ashline D, Dhitavat S, et al. Folate deprivation induces neurodegeneration: roles of oxidative stress and increased homocysteine. *Neurobiol Dis* 2003;14:32-42.

351. Ho PI, Collins SC, Dhitavat S, et al. Homocysteine potentiates beta-amyloid neurotoxicity: role of oxidative stress. *J Neurochem* 2001;78:249-253.

352. Kruman II, Kumaravel TS, Lohani A, et al. Folic acid deficiency and homocysteine impair DNA repair in hippocampal neurons and sensitize them to amyloid toxicity in experimental models of Alzheimer's disease. *J Neurosci* 2002;22:1752-1762.

353. Pak KJ, Chan SL, Mattson MP. Homocysteine and folate deficiency sensitize oligodendrocytes to the cell death-promoting effects of a presenilin-1 mutation and amyloid β-peptide. *Neuromolecular Med* 2003;3:119-128.

354. Courtemanche C, Huang AC, Elson-Schwab I, Kerry N, Ng BY, Ames BN. Folate deficiency and ionizing radiation cause DNA breaks in primary human lymphocytes: a comparison. *FASEB J* 2004;18:209-211.

355. Duan W, Ladenheim B, Cutler RG, Kruman II, Cadet JL, Mattson MP. Dietary folate deficiency and elevated homocysteine levels endanger dopaminergic neurons in models of Parkinson's disease. *J Neurochem* 2002;80:101-110.

356. Kruman II, Culmsee C, Chan SL, et al. Homocysteine elicits a DNA damage response in neurons that promotes apoptosis and hypersensitivity to excitotoxicity. *J Neurosci* 2000;20:6920-6926.

357. Mattson MP, Shea TB. Folate and homocysteine metabolism in neural plasticity and neurodegenerative disorders. *Trends Neurosci* 2003;26:137-146.

358. Kim J, Lee H, Chang N. Hyperhomocysteinemia due to short-term folate deprivation is related to electron microscopic changes in the rat brain. *J Nutr* 2002;132:3418-3421.

359. Fassbender K, Mielke O, Bertsch T, Nafe B, Froschen S, Hennerici M. Homocysteine in cerebral macroangiography and microangiopathy. *Lancet* 1999;353:1586-1587.

360. Hirata S, Matsubara T, Saura R, Tateishi H, Hirohata K. Inhibition of in vitro vascular endothelial cell proliferation and in vivo neovascularization by low-dose methotrexate. *Arthritis Rheum* 1989;32:1065-1073.

361. Joussen AM, Kruse FE, Völcker HE, Kirchhof B. Topical application of methotrexate for inhibition of corneal angiogenesis. *Graefes Arch Clin Exp Ophthalmol* 1999;237:920-927.

362. Mudd SH, Levy HL, Skovby F. Disorders of transsulfuration. In: Scriver CR, Beaudet AL, Sly WS, Valle D, eds. *The metabolic basis of inherited disease.* New York City: McGraw-Hill, 1995:1279-1327.

363. Haworth JC, Dilling LA, Surtees RA, et al. Symptomatic and asymptomatic methylenetetrahydrofolate reductase deficiency in two adult brothers. *Am J Med Genet* 1993;45:572-576.

364. Campbell KCM, Meech RP, Rybak LP, Hughes LF. D-Methionine protects against cisplatin damage to the stria vascularis. *Hear Res* 1999;138:13-28.

365. Campbell KCM, Rybak LP, Meech RP, Hughes L. D-methionine provides excellent protection from cisplatin ototoxicity in the rat. *Hear Res* 1996;102:90-98.

366. Piper MD, Hong SP, Ball GE, Dawes IW. Regulation of the balance of one-carbon metabolism in *Saccharomyces cerevisiae. J Biol Chem* 2000;275:30987-30995.

367. Blood: erythropoiesis - role of folate and vitamin B_{12}. In: Thomas JH, Gillham B, eds. *Wills' Biochemical Basis of Medicine.* 2nd edition. Oxford: Butterworth-Heinemann, 1989:285-296.

368. Ames BN. Mitochondrial decay, a major cause of aging, can be delayed. *J Alzheimers Dis* 2004;6:117-121.

369. Herbig K, Chiang E-P, Lee L-R, Hills J, Shane B, Stover PJ. Cytoplasmic serine hydroxymethyltransferase mediates competition between folate-dependent deoxyribonucleotide and *S*-adenosylmethionine biosyntheses. *J Biol Chem* 2002;277:38381-38389.

370. Girgis S, Suh JR, Jolivet J, Stover PJ. 5-formyltetrahydrofolate regulates homocysteine remethylation in human neuroblastoma. *J Biol Chem* 1997;272:4729-4734.

371. Elverland HH, Torbergsen T. Audiologic findings in a family with mitochondrial disorder. *Am J Otol* 1991;12:459-465.

372. Sergi B, Ferraresi A, Troiani D, Paludetti G, Fetoni AR. Cisplatin ototoxicity in the guinea pig: vestibular and cochlear damage. *Hear Res* 2003;182:56-64.

373. Kopelman J, Budnick AS, Sessions RB, Kramer MB, Wong GY. Ototoxicity of high-dose cisplatin by bolus administration in patients with advanced cancers and normal hearing. *Laryngoscope* 1988;98:858-864.

374. Kruidering M, Van de Water B, de Heer E, Mulder GJ, Nagelkerke JF. Cisplatin-induced nephrotoxicity in porcine proximal tubular cells: mitochondrial dysfunction by inhibition of complexes I to IV of the respiratory chain. *J Pharmacol Exp Ther* 1997;280:638-649.

375. Kim J-S, Shane B. Role of folylpolyglutamate synthetase in the metabolism and cytotoxicity of 5-deazaacyclotetrahydrofolate, an anti-purine drug. *J Biol Chem* 1994;269:9714-9720.

Summary

Folate and age-related disease

Demographic trends show that by 2050, approximately 30% of people in industrialized countries will be 65 years or older. Aging is associated with increased risk of cardiovascular and neurodegenerative disorders and increased prevalence of their risk factors. Slowing down age-related disease processes will add quality to longer lives and should be an imperative for public health policy. Modifiable risk factors for age-related diseases need to be identified and their causality determined. The prevalence of low concentrations of folate and high concentrations of homocysteine in the blood increases with age, perhaps in part as a consequence to changes in dietary pattern. Both low folate and high homocysteine concentrations have been associated with cardiovascular disease and neurodegenerative disorders. Homocysteine is an amino acid located at the fork of two pathways in the metabolism of methionine, which relies on coenzymes derived from vitamin B_{12}, folate and vitamin B_6. The majority of hyperhomocysteinemic cases are attributed to low B vitamin levels. In addition, a 677C→T mutation in the gene encoding 5,10-methylenetetrahydrofolate reductase (MTHFR), a key enzyme in the remethylation cycle, increases homocysteine by approximately 25% in subjects with the MTHFR 677TT genotype. Supplementation with folic acid can reduce homocysteine concentrations by approximately 25% in the general population.

We investigated the association of folate and homocysteine with risk of cardiovascular disease, as measured by carotid intima-media thickness and arterial stiffness (Chapter 3), cognitive performance (Chapter 4) and hearing (Chapter 5). Cross-sectional data come from the participants of the FACIT trial obtained from the baseline measurements. FACIT is an acronym for Folic Acid and Carotid Intima-media Thickness. The FACIT trial investigates the effects of 0.8 mg folic acid supplementation for three years on carotid intima-media thickness, cognitive function and hearing in 819 middle-aged and elderly Dutch men and women. In addition, we investigated the effect of one-year folic acid supplementation on inflammation markers (Chapter 6). Inflammation is the initial step in the atherosclerotic process and has been associated with cardiovascular disease, dementia and hearing loss.

Symptomatic vascular disease is preceded by atherosclerotic changes in the arterial system and is culminated by triggers such as plaque disruption and secondary thrombotic complications leading to vessel occlusion and subsequent ischemia. Carotid intima-media thickness is a valid surrogate marker of vascular disease and a marker of generalized atherosclerosis. Whether low folate or high homocysteine concentrations exert their effects via thrombotic or atherogenic mechanisms and whether they are involved in early or advanced stages of atherosclerosis is uncertain. In the 819 FACIT participants, low concentrations of erythrocyte folate were associated with increased carotid intima-media thickness, independent of other vascular disease risk factors (mean difference first vs. third quartile 0.03 mm, 95% CI 0.004 to 0.06 mm, first vs. fourth quartile 0.03 mm, 95% CI -0.002 to 0.06 mm). Homocysteine, on the other hand, was not associated with carotid intima-media thickness. In contrast to carotid intima-media thickness, neither folate nor homocysteine were associated with carotid distension, a marker of arterial stiffness. Our findings support a pathogenic role of low folate in atherosclerosis and vascular disease, through mechanisms other than homocysteine-lowering. We were the first research group to detect an inverse association between folate and carotid intima-media thickness, perhaps because other study populations had an adequate folate status.

Low folate concentrations, hyperhomocysteinemia and vascular disease have been implicated in poor cognitive performance. We investigated whether folate was associated with cognitive performance using a battery of cognitive tests sensitive to age-related cognitive decline. In addition, we explored whether the association of folate with cognitive function was independent of homocysteine and vascular disease. Low concentrations of folate were associated to poor cognitive performance on memory and speed-related functions, independent of vascular disease and its risk factors, including homocysteine. Our results support a role of folate in age-related cognitive decline, as tests performed poorly by subjects with low folate concentrations were the same tests with the greatest variability with age. Although low folate and high homocysteine were associated with poor cognitive performance, the MTHFR 677TT genotype was associated with better cognitive function. Given the small sample size of our population, the protective association observed with the MTHFR 677TT genotype and better cognitive performance may be due to chance. However, if our findings are confirmed in larger study populations, this may implicate the other phenotypic differences related to MTHFR 677TT genotype, besides increased homocysteine concentrations. For example, subjects with the MTHFR 677TT genotype may experience a shift in the folate derivative distribution, favoring formyl-folate derivatives and possibly favoring formyl-folate driven reactions such as *de novo* nucleotide synthesis and mitochondrial oxidative phosphorylation. Both of these processes may be important for DNA fidelity and mitochondrial health of the neuron.

Age-related hearing loss is one of the four most common disorders of the elderly. Despite studies that observed cochlear deformations in animals fed diets deficient in B vitamins, little attention has been given to the role of diet, including folate, in the prevalence or incidence of age-related hearing loss. We investigated the association of folate with hearing thresholds in 729 participants with age-related hearing loss from the FACIT trial. Contrary to our *a priori* hypothesis, folate, not homocysteine, was directly associated with hearing impairment. Researchers have speculated that the activity of the enzymes involved in folate metabolism depend in part on intracellular folate concentrations. Specifically, low folate concentrations may mimic the MTHFR 677TT genotype, such that a greater competition exists favoring formyl-folate reactions, which then may enhance DNA stability and oxidative mitochondrial phosphorylation. In fact, subjects with the MTHFR 677TT genotype had better hearing than subjects with the CC or CT genotype and low folate concentrations were associated with poorer hearing in subjects with the MTHFR 677C allele only. If our findings are confirmed in other populations, then more research should be conducted on the role of formyl-folates in relation to cochlear health and hearing.

Low folate and high homocysteine concentrations have been associated with a proinflammatory state. Inflammation, on the other hand, has been associated with vascular disease and dementia. We investigated the effect of one-year folic acid supplementation and subsequent homocysteine-lowering on inflammation markers in middle-aged and elderly men and women. A randomized controlled trial design was used to evaluate the effect of one-year folic acid treatment on plasma concentrations of oxidized low-density lipoprotein (LDL), autoantibodies against oxidized LDL, soluble intercellular adhesion molecule-1 and C-reactive protein in the final 530 subjects enrolled in the FACIT trial. Although folic acid supplementation caused a considerable increase in serum folate (430% increase) and a reduction in homocysteine (25% decrease) concentrations, we found no decrease in plasma concentrations of the inflammation markers. The pathogenic mechanism associated with low folate and high homocysteine concentrations remains elusive. Low concentrations of folate and high concentrations of homocysteine may affect cardiovascular risk through other oxidative or inflammatory mechanisms or through hemostasis. However, in a sub-sample of FACIT participants we have shown that one-year folic acid supplementation did not affect markers in the hemostasis or fibrinolytic pathways.

In summary, we have found that low concentrations of folate are associated with increased carotid intima-media thickness, a marker of cardiovascular disease risk and poor cognitive performance. Contrary to our expectations, low concentrations of folate were associated with hearing acuity, although this was confined to subjects with the MTHFR 677C allele. In agreement with previous studies, homocysteine was not associated with carotid intima-media thickness, arterial stiffness and hearing levels, but was associated with various tests of cognitive function. Oxidized LDL, autoantibodies against oxidized LDL, C-reactive protein and soluble intercellular adhesion molecule-1, all markers of inflammation, are not affected by folic acid supplementation. Although observational epidemiology has led to much optimism for folate as a panacea for age-related diseases such as cardiovascular disease and neurodegenerative disorders, it is prudent for public health policy makers to await trials—the conventional golden standard by which to test causality—before deciding on folic acid fortification for the general population.

Samenvatting

Folaat en ouderdomsziekten

Demografische trends voorspellen dat in 2050 ongeveer 30% van de bevolking in geïndustrialiseerde landen 65 jaar of ouder zal zijn. Ouder worden gaat gepaard met een toenemende kans op hart- en vaatziekten, aandoeningen van het zenuwstelsel en een toenemende prevalentie van risicofactoren voor deze ziekten. Het vertragen van de processen die leiden tot ouderdomsziekten kan zorgen voor een langer en kwalitatief beter leven en zou daarom een belangrijk aandachtspunt voor overheidsbeleid moeten zijn. Risicofactoren die beïnvloed kunnen worden door voeding en andere leefstijlfactoren moeten daartoe geïdentificeerd worden, bijvoorbeeld met behulp van epidemiologisch onderzoek. Vervolgens moet worden vastgesteld of het om oorzakelijke relaties gaat. De prevalentie van lage concentraties van folaat, een B vitamine, en daarmee hoge concentraties van homocysteïne in het bloed neemt toe met het ouder worden, en dit kan mede komen door een veranderd voedingspatroon bij veroudering. Zowel een lage folaatstatus als een hoge homocysteïne concentratie hangen samen met een verhoogde kans op hart- en vaatziekten en aandoeningen van het zenuwstelsel. Homocysteïne is een aminozuur dat een belangrijke schakel is in het metabolisme van methionine. Het homocysteïne gehalte is afhankelijk van de co-enzymen vitamine B_{12}, folaat en vitamine B_6. De meerderheid van de hyperhomocysteïnemische gevallen is toe te schrijven aan lage vitamine B concentraties. Bovendien verhoogt de 677C$\rightarrow$T mutatie in het gen dat codeert voor 5,10-methyleentetrahydrofolaat reductase (MTHFR), een sleutelenzym in de remethylering van homocysteïne naar methionine, het homocysteïnegehalte met gemiddeld 25% bij mensen met het MTHFR 677TT genotype. Suppletie met foliumzuur (de synthetische vorm van folaat) kan het homocysteïne gehalte met gemiddeld 25% verlagen in de algemene bevolking.

In dit proefschrift is het verband onderzocht tussen folaatstatus en homocysteïne enerzijds en de kans op hart- en vaatziekten (Hoofdstuk 3), cognitief functioneren (Hoofdstuk 4) en gehoor (Hoofdstuk 5) anderzijds. Risico op hart- en vaatziekten werd geschat via het echografisch meten van de stijfheid en dikte van de wand van de halsslagader. De cross-sectionele data betreffen de eerste (baseline) metingen van de deelnemers aan het FACIT-onderzoek. FACIT staat voor *Folic Acid and Carotid Intima-media Thickness.* Het FACIT-onderzoek is een gerandomiseerd, placebo-gecontroleerd onderzoek naar de effecten van suppletie met 0,8 mg foliumzuur gedurende drie jaar op de dikte van de halsslagader, het cognitief functioneren en gehoor bij 819 Nederlandse mannen en vrouwen in de leeftijd van 50 tot 70 jaar. Deze studie zal halverwege 2005 de einddata rapporteren. In een subgroep is het effect onderzocht van een jaar foliumzuursuppletie op ontstekingsmarkers (Hoofdstuk 6). Ontsteking is de eerste stap in het ontstaan van slagaderverkalking of arteriosclerose en is geassocieerd met hart- en vaatziekten, dementie en gehoorverlies.

Symptomatische vaatziekten worden vaak vooraf gegaan door arteriosclerotische veranderingen in de bloedvaten. Een hart- of herseninfarct wordt veroorzaakt door de afsluiting van een bloedvat als gevolg van losgekomen bloedproppen of plaatselijke trombosevorming. De dikte van de halsslagader is een valide marker voor hart- en vaatziekten: het voorspelt de kans op een hart- of herseninfarct. Het is onzeker of een lage folaat of een hoge homocysteïne concentratie werkelijk een oorzaak zijn van hart- en vaatziekten. Verder is onduidelijk of het effect loopt via processen van trombose of aderverkalking, en in welke fase van bloedvatvernauwing dan precies. Bij de 819 FACIT deelnemers waren lage concentraties van folaat in de rode bloedcellen geassocieerd met een dikkere wand van de halsslagader, onafhankelijk van andere risicofactoren van hart en vaatziekten (gemiddeld verschil tussen het eerste en derde kwartiel 0,03 mm, 95% betrouwbaarheidsinterval 0,004 tot 0,06 mm; gemiddeld verschil tussen het eerste en vierde kwartiel 0,03 mm, 95% betrouwbaarheidsinterval -0,002 tot 0,06 mm). Homocysteïne was niet gerelateerd aan de dikte van de halsslagaderwand. Zowel folaat als homocysteïne waren niet geassocieerd met distensie van de halsslagader, een indicator voor de rekbaarheid van bloedvaten. Onze bevindingen steunen de veronderstelling dat een laag folaatgehalte een rol speelt bij het ontstaan van arteriosclerose en vaatziekten, maar wel via andere mechanismen dan het verhogen van het homocysteïnegehalte. Wij zijn de eerste onderzoeksgroep die een omgekeerd verband vonden tussen folaat en de dikte van de halsslagader, waarschijnlijk doordat andere onderzoekspopulaties een adequate folaatstatus hadden.

Een lage folaatconcentratie, hyperhomocysteïnemie en vaatziekten zijn factoren die bijdragen aan slecht cognitief functioneren. We hebben onderzocht of folaat geassocieerd is met cognitief functioneren. Hierbij hebben we gebruik gemaakt van een aantal testen die een afname in de aan veroudering gerelateerde cognitieve functies kunnen meten. Daarnaast hebben we gekeken of het verband tussen folaat en cognitief functioneren onafhankelijk is van homocysteïne en vaatziekten. Lage concentraties folaat waren geassocieerd met een slechte score op cognitief functioneren, op het gebied van geheugen en snelheid van cognitieve processen. Dit was onafhankelijk van vaatziekten en hun risicofactoren, inclusief homocysteïne. Onze bevindingen ondersteunen dat folaat een rol speelt bij cognitieve functies bij ouderen. Hoewel lage folaat en hoge homocysteïne concentraties geassocieerd waren met slechtere cognitieve functie, was het MTHFR 677TT genotype geassocieerd met een betere cognitieve functie. Door het relatief kleine aantal deelnemers in onze studie kan dit positieve verband tussen het MTHFR 677TT genotype en het beter cognitieve functioneren ook op een statistisch toeval berusten. Maar als onze bevindingen kunnen worden bevestigd in een grotere studiepopulatie zou een eventuele verklaring kunnen liggen in andere fenotypische verschillen bij het MTHFR 677TT genotype. Zo zouden bijvoorbeeld mensen met een MTHFR 677TT genotype een verschuiving in hun routes van folaatmetabolisme kunnen hebben ten gunste van formyl-folaat derivativen. Hierdoor zouden formyl-folaat gestuurde reacties als *de novo* nucleotidesynthese en mitochondriale oxidatieve phosphorylering beter kunnen verlopen. Beide processen kunnen belangrijk zijn voor de DNA conditie en de mitochondriale conditie van een neuron.

Gehoorverlies is een belangrijke ouderdomskwaal. Ondanks het feit dat studies bij dieren hebben aangetoond dat vitamine B deficiënte diëten leiden tot vervormingen in het binnenoor, is er nauwelijks aandacht voor de rol van voedingspatronen, inclusief folaat inname, bij het ontstaan van gehoorverlies bij ouderen. We hebben het verband onderzocht tussen folaat en gehoordrempels (het aantal decibels waarbij men een toon nog net hoort) bij 729 deelnemers met een aan ouderdom gerelateerd gehoorverlies binnen het FACIT-onderzoek. In tegenstelling tot onze veronderstelde hypothese bleek dat een lage folaatstatus gepaard ging met een beter gehoor, maar alleen in de groep met het MTHFR 677C allel. Homocysteïne hing niet samen met gehoor. Daarnaast hadden deelnemers met een MTFHR 677TT genotype een beter gehoor dan respondenten met een CC of CT genotype. Lage folaatconcentraties zouden kunnen leiden tot een situatie die vergelijkbaar is met het MTHFR 677TT genotype, waarbij er meer formyl-folaat reacties plaatsvinden. Deze reacties kunnen de DNA stabiliteit en de mitochondriale conditie versterken. Als onze bevindingen worden bevestigd in andere populaties dan zou er meer onderzoek gedaan moeten worden naar de rol van formyl-folaat in relatie tot de gezondheid van het binnenoor en het gehoor.

Lage folaat en hoge homocysteïne concentraties zijn geassocieerd met een verhoogde kans op ontstekingen, welke als mogelijke oorzaak van hart- en vaatziekten en dementie worden gezien. In het gerandomiseerde, placebo-gecontroleerde FACIT-onderzoek is eveneens onderzocht wat de effecten zijn van één jaar suppletie met foliumzuur op ontstekingsindicatoren bij 530 mannen en vrouwen tussen de 50 en 70 jaar. De onderzochte markers waren geoxideerde lage-dichtheidslipoproteïne deeltjes, immunoglobuline G antilichamen en immunoglobuline M antilichamen tegen geoxideerde lage-dichtheidslipoproteïne deeltjes, circulerend intercellulair adhesie eiwit-1 en C-reactieve proteïne. Hoewel de foliumzuursuppletie zorgde voor een aanzienlijke toename van het serumfolaat (een toename van 430%) en een afname van het homocysteïne gehalte (een afname van 25%), vonden we geen afname van de plasmaconcentraties van de ontstekingsindicatoren. Dit hoeft nog niet te betekenen dat extra foliumzuur geen bescherming tegen hart- en vaatziekten biedt, want het zou via heel andere mechanismen kunnen verlopen.

Samengevat kan gesteld worden dat lage concentraties folaat geassocieerd zijn met een toename van de intima-media dikte van de halsslagader, een indicator voor een verhoogd risico van hart- en vaatziekten, en een slechter cognitief functioneren. Anders dan we verwacht hadden, leidden lage concentraties folaat tot een scherper gehoor. Dit was wel beperkt tot de groep met een MTFHR 677C allel. In overeenstemming met voorgaande onderzoeken was homocysteïne niet geassocieerd met de intima-media dikte van de halsslagader, stijfheid van de halsslagader of gehoor, maar wel met diverse cognitieve functie testen. Indicatoren van ontstekingen werden niet beïnvloed door foliumzuursuppletie. Hoewel observationele studies hebben geleid tot een groot optimisme voor folaat als het wondermiddel voor ouderdomsziekten, is het zeer verstandig om te wachten op experimenteel onderzoek—de gewone gouden standaard waarin causaliteit vastgesteld wordt—voordat er besloten wordt tot verrijking van voedsel met foliumzuur voor de gehele populatie.

Acknowledgements

It is my great pleasure to acknowledge the many whom have contributed to the research described in this thesis. First I would like to thank the people who were interested in participating in the FACIT study. It is your altruistic mindset that will cast long shadows on evidence-based public health policy. Of the thousands who were willing to participate, I would like to thank the 819 FACIT study participants who had loyally taken their allocated treatment and attended the laborious and quite personal measurement sessions at the Wageningen University. Thank you, for your perseverance and enthusiasm.

My hat goes off to the FACIT team. Such a large and busy study is not your everyday job and requires motivation and dedication, flexiblility, being a team player, precision and active communication skills. Once started, the FACIT study was like a train on which you had to jump or get run over. Even in the Dutch flatlands, the FACIT train took us to the proverbial peaks and valleys. Nevertheless, your enthusiasm and friendliness made the social extras possible such as eel fishing, pottery throwing, a lot of good eatin' and vacation photo evenings. Your enthusiasm, without a doubt, creeped into the FACIT study and stimulated and maintained the professional extras such as a loaded FACIT study bag, an impressive FACIT Family Day, birthday and Christmas cards, "Folaatgepraat" and the Big Band party to celebrate 1.5 years of FACIT with the study participants. Thanks for making the FACIT study more than just a job. Thanks for doing it so well. Thanks for doing it all!

I would like to thank Josette van As and Ondine van de Rest for doing a fantastic job organizing the FACIT screening phase and the FACIT study phase, respectively. Marga van der Steen was responsible for the detailed blood protocol, the careful preparation of the blood and many other aspects important for sample administration and tracking. I would like to thank her and the research assistants—Anita Willebrand, Henny Krielaart, Elly Monster, Trudy Jansen, Anja ter Haar, Charlotte Rijsemus, Els van der Ven, Lucy Okma—for the blood quickly taken from hundreds of hungry, sleepy study participants early in the morning. I would like to thank Liesbeth Smeets and Jantien Takens for their excellent work on the ultrasound machine and the many hearing and cognitive tests which they have conducted. Many others have done valuable tasks within the FACIT study over the past five years. I would like to thank Marieke Verheijden, Marieke Nijmeijer, Janette de Goede, Gea Schouten, Halime Ozturk, Joke Benjamins, Annemarie Voortman, Gerda Pot, Siska van der Laan and Liselore van Nunen. Last but not least, undergraduate students have contributed to the FACIT study, though unfortunately unpaid. They assisted in fieldwork, data entry, and many communication tasks alongside analyzing data from the FACIT study and presenting their findings in written and oral form. Without Halime Ozturk's dedication, Carla Enthoven's independence, Grea van Wijngaarden's politeness, Huang Du's diligence, Eunice Gonçalves nonchalance and Karin Haks' and Winette van den Brandhof's creativity, the FACIT study would have been paler.

The other FACIT team—my co-promotor and promoters—I would like to thank, foremost Petra Verhoef. I have really grown under Petra's regimen of creativity and freedom and have immensely enjoyed working with her. Petra was responsible for the creation of the FACIT study—writing up the study proposal and securing funds—and has actively taken part making the FACIT study a success. I have learned from and appreciated Evert Schouten's openness and well-weighed comments on the conduct of the FACIT research and on our papers. In addition, I will fondly remember our funny moments together (e.g. metro in Milan). Speaking about funny moments, I have enjoyed working with Frans Kok and, of course, on a more critical note, have benefited from his bird's eye view of a paper and project. Thanks for all that I have learned under your supervision; it has been a lot of fun working together with all of you.

I would like to thank the co-authors for their contribution to the methodology of the FACIT study and their critical comments on the manuscripts. Several have ensured that our collaboration was a success. We have enjoyed the training from and the collaboration with Michiel Bots, Rick Grobbee, Rudy Meijer, Frank Leus, Frances Verheij, Dicky Mooiweer, Karin Nijssen and Annemarie Rijswijk of Julius Center for Health Sciences and Primary Care and Lucien Anteunis, Martin van Boxtel, Astrid Quist and Carlein Karimoen of Brain and Behavior Institute. Finally, our collaboration with Berry van Tits and Heidi Hak of Univesity Medical Center Nijmegen was fruitful and enjoyable.

I would like to thank the many laboratories which have timely analyzed hundreds of our samples: Dorine Swinkels and Siem Klaver from Radboud University Nijmegen; Ton Teerlink from Open University; Gijs de Kort and Paul Franck from the hematology department at Leyenburg Hospital, Eric Huetink from Velp hospital; and Jan Harryvan, Tineke van Roekel, Dennis Snoeck, Paul Hulshof and the late Peter van Bovenkamp from Wageningen University. Related to all of our biochemical analyses, I would like to thank Pieter Versloot for assistance with the blood label program; Dick van Rumpt and

Harry Schonewille from SHO for providing personnel to conduct venipunctures; and Pieter Versteeg and Ad Budding for transporting the blood and ultrasound tapes to their various destinations.

Many people from the division of Human Nutrition have helped make sure that the FACIT study was a success. I would like to thank Marie Jansen for answering stray telephone calls and for sifting through all of the post we generated; Riekie Janssen and Eric van Munster for all of the financial administrative help; Ben Scholte, Anne Baars and the late Dirk Joghems for curing my computer pains; Dione Bouchaut for technical assistance with "Folaatgepraat;" Joke Barendse for help screening logistics; Lidwien van der Heyden for handling all of our personnel administration; Els Siebelink for organizing all of the breakfasts; and Saskia Meyboom and Petra Vissink for help with blinding. Finally, it has been a pleasure to have the opportunity to work together with other members of the division to include new markers in the FACIT study. Mariska Klerk was responsible for hemostasis markers, Margreet Olthof for carotid plaque measurements and Marielle Engberink, together with Marianne Geleijnse, Wim de Kort and Dorine Swinkels, for iron markers.

Also, many people not in our division have contributed to the FACIT study for which I am grateful. I would like to thank Wim de Kort from Nijmegen Bloedbank for his generous help with recruitment; Huub Willems for the randomization lists; Beitske and Marianne Stoelinga for making the information session video (just in case participants didn't understand my Dutch!); the baker, Mr. van Woerekom, for allowing us to give the study participants a piece of cake with a cup of coffee; Jan van der Roest from SwissCaps for supplying us with folic acid and placebo capsules; Sandra Bausch, Henny Brants and Marco Bouman from TNO for developing our folate food frequency questionnaire; Gert-Jan Kloos for developing our ideal database; Aly van Loenen for the handmade birthday cards; and Kweekvijver and Tweedee for the creation and maintenance of the FACIT internet site (www.facit.net), respectively. Finally, I would like to thank Sanne Schuts, from Sanne Schuts Ontwerpen for the cover design of this book and Ray Edgar for capturing such a nice glimpse of Nature on film.

Alongside the research monies granted from ZonMw and Wageningen University, I am grateful for the generous financial support from Wageningen Centre for Food Sciences for the FACIT study and for my own studies at Netherlands Institute for Health Sciences. I would also like to thank Martijn Katan, Els van den Worm, Edith

Bodegraven and Hannie van Oosten from WCFS for their scientific, administrative and technical support.

Alongside my education, I have prospered in many ways while conducting my doctorate research in Wageningen. My many thanks go to my colleagues at the Division of Human Nutrition for making my time there with you so enjoyable. Finally, I would like to thank the ever-changing group on the sixth floor for all of the discussions, laughs, cake, filthy coffee cups and dinners. I thank the many clubs of which I was a member for their constructive feedback. I would like to thank my paranymphs for helping organize the festivities that will take place after my graduation and for selective proofreading. Finally, I would like to thank the late Clive West for sending me to the European Nutrition Leadership Programme and for his lively and comforting discussions.

Even people not officially involved in nutrition research have helped make the FACIT study such a success, and that is my family. Thank you, my loving, supportive family, for all of the years of patience and interest for the activities of such an absent-minded daughter, sister, wife and mother. The least I can do is give this to you in return.

JANE DURGA WAS born on April 23, 1973 in Heidelberg, Germany and grew-up in Germany and the United States of America. In 1991, she went to India for her final year of high school as a Rotary exchange student (St. Xavier's College, Bombay). On her return to the United States of America, she enrolled in the General Sciences program at Northwestern Michigan College. In 1993 she received her Associate's degree with Honors. After receiving the Harry S. Truman Scholarship in 1993, a scholarship which finances undergraduate and graduate studies for students with leadership potential and a commitment to a career in public service. Thus, rather than work during the summer, Jane volunteered in Matagalpa, Nicaragua at a high-risk pregnancy shelter, doing everything from aerobics to yoga with highly pregnant women. In 1994, she joined a United States of America / European Union initiative, which allowed her to complete her undergraduate degree at University of Aberdeen (*Environmental Microbiology*) in combination with Michigan State University (*BSc Microbiology with Honors, 1995*). During her undergraduate studies Jane worked as a sexual health educator and served on the HIV Prevention and Planning Commission for the Department of Public Health, State of Michigan. In the summer of 1995, she contributed to a national review of environmental toxins by the National Center for Environmental Assessment, United States Environmental Protection Agency in Washington DC. In the fall of that year, she received a postgraduate Rotary scholarship and moved to the tropical and spicy island of Zanzibar, Tanzania to enroll in Kiswahili courses. With her newly learned Kiswahili, she enrolled later that year in the postgraduate Parasitology program of Moi University in Eldoret, Kenya. In an attempt to try work outside a laboratory, she studied human nutrition at the London School of Hygiene and Tropical Medicine in the United Kingdom (*MSc Human Nutrition, 1997*).

Jane moved to The Netherlands in 1997 where she worked on both urban nutrition and household food security at the Royal Tropical Institute in Amsterdam and on nutrition and meal composition at KLM Airlines in Schipol. In 1999 she joined the Human Nutrition Division at Wageningen University. There she worked under the supervision of Petra Verhoef on a large randomized controlled trial as part of her PhD project. During her doctorate training, Jane attended the Netherlands Institute of Health Sciences (*MSc Epidemiology, 2003*) and the European Nutrition Leadership Programme. Jane continues her work in the field of folate at the Human Nutrition Division as a post-doc fellow. She lives with her husband, Bendrie, and son, Jasper, in a typical Dutch *rijtje* house in Wageningen, The Netherlands.

Training and supervision

NWO Voeding, 1999-2001, 2003

WUR PhD Excursion, South Africa, Switzerland, Germany, Italy, 1999, 2001

WEON, Dutch Epidemiology Society, 2000, 2001, 2003

Food Summit, Wageningen Centre for Food Sciences, 2001

Third & Fourth International Conference on Homocysteine Metabolism, 2001, 2003

Dutch Endo-Neuro-Psych Conference, 2002, 2004

Third Conference on Hyperhomocysteinemia, 2003

Type 2 Diabetes Mellitus: Causes, Consequences and Therapy, VLAG, 2003

Systematic Literature Research, VLAG, 2003

Brain and Cognition Symposium, University of Maastricht, 2003, 2004

First International Congress on Geriatric/Gerontologic Audiology, 2004

European Nutrition Leadership Programme, 2004

Sixth Vascular Biology Workshop, University Hospital Maastricht, 2004

FASEB Folic acid, Vitamin B_{12} & One-carbon Metabolism, 2004

Netherlands Institute for Health Sciences, *MSc Epidemiology*, 2000-2003

The research described in this thesis was funded by a grant from the Netherlands Organisation for Health Research and Development (ZonMw, grant number 20010002), Wageningen Centre for Food Sciences and Wageningen University.

Financial support for the publication of this thesis by the Wageningen University and Wageningen Centre for Food Sciences is gratefully acknowledged.

Cover photography: Ray Edgar, Carmanthenshire, United Kingdom
Cover design: Sanne Schuts Ontwerpen, The Hague, The Netherlands
Printing: Ponsen & Looijen, Wageningen, The Netherlands